Your Sleep Story

Your Sleep Story

A NO-HYPE GUIDE TO SLEEP HEALTH

Matt Bianchi MD, PhD

This book is provided for informational purposes only and is not meant to be exhaustive. References to selected publications and web sites are provided as additional sources for the interested reader, but do not represent an endorsement of any views, advice, products or services referenced there. The content is not intended to represent or replace the advice of a trained professional, does not establish a doctor-patient relationship and should not be used to diagnose or treat a disease or medical condition. As with any source of information about health, seek the counsel of a trained professional for any questions or concerns you may have.
The content of this book is designed to be general, drawing from common themes over years of clinical experience. Any similarities to actual patients or conversations are coincidental.

Editorial support by CreateSpace and Balaji Goparaju.
Cover by www.99designs.com designer Andi (adr98) and Vera Bevini.

ISBN-13: 9781979731799
ISBN-10: 1979731799

To my patients, for teaching me more about sleep than any textbook ever could.

Contents

How to read this book

Welcome! Because each chapter in this book is designed to stand alone, you can read the book in any order, if a particular chapter title sounds most relevant to you after a quick glance at the table of contents. Or you can just read it in order, like a regular book. I focused the content on common topics in sleep health for adults. In each chapter, you'll find suggestions (mainly as footnotes) to visit other parts of the book for related information. This is not just a throwback to how much I enjoyed childhood "Choose Your Own Adventure" books—it's an homage to every patient I've ever seen in my sleep clinic, where clues and context always take us on decision-making turns both expected and unexpected. References are provided as superscript numbers throughout the text, as much to back up statements and ideas as to offer suggestions for those who want to dig a little deeper (and where the articles are open access, the URL is provided in the reference section at the end of the book).

Here's what this book is not: miracle cures, revolutionary secrets, and shocking claims. Some people find these approaches highly motivating, but in my clinical experience, these approaches don't sit well with how I talk to my patients, so I can't make them sit well in the pages of my book. This book was inspired by the privilege I've had to care for thousands of patients with sleep problems, and I wouldn't put anything to paper that I wouldn't say in a clinical visit or behind a lecture podium.

CHAPTER 1

Start here (or any other chapter)

You'd expect the experts to agree

Sleep is not supposed to be a controversial field. We might not understand all the magic and mystery of sleep, and we might not always give sleep the highest priority in our busy lives. But it's not like the experts are arguing about sleep and health, right? Hearing about research proclaiming that sleep is important for this or that aspect of health more often triggers an "of course—we knew that" response, or even a bored yawn, rather than a response of skepticism.

We shouldn't let the appearance of obviousness, or common repetition in the media, lull us into complacency. We'll look at a few examples in this chapter to give you a flavor of some of the surprising disagreements the experts have among themselves. I'm not talking about digging into obscure corners of academic libraries for creative naysayers and pessimists; I'm talking about finding controversy and uncertainty in the medical literature version of "broad daylight." Throughout the book we'll need to navigate uncertainty: not simply as a mental exercise but because we have to make real-world decisions about our sleep—and about our health in general—with often-incomplete information. Just as we need to balance risks and benefits in our own personal decisions, my goal is to balance uncertainty in the science of sleep medicine. When we think that the experts are in agreement, we may place too much confidence or acceptance on generalities that may not apply to us as individuals. When we focus too much on the disagreements, we may feel cynical and place too little confidence in the science.

One recent example appeared in 2016 in the prestigious *New England Journal of Medicine*: treating obstructive sleep apnea did not prevent heart attacks in a large multinational research study.[1] This was a bombshell for a sleep medicine field that has been working hard to improve the diagnosis and treatment of sleep apnea in part to improve heart health. How should we think about this finding? Is it possible that sleep medicine doctors have fundamentally misunderstood the health risks of sleep apnea? That seems unlikely, considering the several decades' worth of research that has linked untreated sleep apnea to heart attacks and strokes and other health risks. Is it possible that something was awry in the research study that compromised the results? This also seems unlikely, since the research involved the international collaboration of top experts and was published in a top medical journal. This is not just a question for academic conferences and journal club discussions. Would primary-care doctors now wonder if this finding were reliable enough to change the way they talked to their patients about sleep apnea? Would patients now wonder if the effort of wearing a mask to treat sleep apnea would be worth it? If we really believe that one of the strongest motivations for treating sleep apnea has been dethroned, would a cloud of skepticism extend to other less-supported sleep research topics?

The fact that findings like this aren't just isolated instances makes it even more important to consider how to deal with this kind of uncertainty. The last few years alone have seen numerous publications that have questioned or contradicted even the most simple-sounding ideas about sleep health. We'll dive into some of these topics in other chapters, but a few stand out for now. In March 2017, the Accreditation Council for Graduate Medical Education, which oversees physician training in America, revised their work-hours regulations,[2] replacing the current rules with the less restrictive 2003 regulations. This decision was based on a review of evidence on the topic, including a large study that reported no patient-safety benefits of the more restrictive work-hours regulations.[3] Obviously nobody wants a sleepy doctor, but the question of work hours policy to improve patient safety turns out to be not so simple.

In April 2017, the American Academy of Sleep Medicine released a statement[4] recommending delayed school start times (the American Academy of Pediatrics had also made this recommendation in 2014). Also in 2017, the prestigious Cochrane Library released a major study (known as a systematic review[5]) that concluded that the evidence in favor of delaying school start times was so limited that the effects could not be determined.

In June 2015, the American Academy of Sleep Medicine released a consensus statement,[6] jointly with the Sleep Research Society, on the recommended amount of sleep for adults: at least 7 hours. While many authorities describe modern society as suffering from an epidemic of sleep loss, an extensive review of research in this area concluded that no significant change to sleep duration has occurred over the past fifty years.[7] If an editorial[8] from 1894 in the *British Medical Journal* is any indication, then blaming widespread insomnia on the pace and anxiety of "modern" life also hasn't changed much over the last century or so.

Perhaps the most controversial discovery of recent years actually resulted in a patient-safety warning: in May 2015, a large multinational clinical trial discovered that a special kind of mask system used to treat "central" and "complex" sleep apnea (which I'll discuss in chapter 11) called adaptive servo-ventilation actually increased the risk of cardiovascular death in some people.[9]

Much has been written about each of these topics, and this is part of the point: experts can disagree with one another, and seemingly well-done research studies can disagree with one other. The debates even include fundamental questions like: What pattern of sleep stages reflects good sleep quality sleep? An expert panel of sleep specialists could not come to a consensus on this question.[10,11] That doesn't mean we lose faith in the process. But if you're thinking about making a decision that could potentially affect your health, or you're developing an opinion about a policy, then the one thing you want to avoid is assuming that the case is already closed.

Forests and trees and Zs

As someone who's spent his entire adult life in academia, I'm painfully familiar with the criticism we academics get all the time that we're so immersed in the details, we often lose the big picture. This can create a gap between the research world—of careful experiments (and jargon-filled publications)—and the real world, which is never quite so neatly arranged as that. Which world is more likely to be relevant for people who are trying to make the best decision about sleep or about their health in general? Each chapter in this book provides suggestions for how to answer this question—because the answer is less about which research study or treatment recommendation is right or wrong in itself and more about how to apply the information in each person's context.

I chose the title "Forests and Trees" for one of the first presentations I made as a graduate student 20 years ago. At the time, I had just started my PhD thesis on how nerve cells communicate with one another using electrical signals. I found myself grappling with the problem of whether it was better to study the tiny openings in a single cell that conduct electricity one channel at a time, or if we should study the entire nerve cell at once. I was so far into the details that a single nerve actually qualified as the big picture, a veritable "forest" of many thousands of channels. My conclusion in favor of studying the individual protein "trees" was less important than my eventual realization that this metaphorical contrast of the forest and the trees applies to many questions. The trick was realizing that what is a forest and what is a tree depends on what scale you're looking at. The people who study even "entire" nerve cells (the forest, to my graduate school self) can seem very detail oriented to those who study brain circuits involving millions of nerve cells, not to mention people who study the ultimate big picture of human behavior.

As I transitioned out of the laboratory and into the hospital, I was immediately struck by two other contrasts. The one that really stopped me in my tracks was the realization that the neurologists who prescribe medications were not using the knowledge of nerve cell electricity to aid their clinical decisions. On the patient wards and in the clinics, this minutia was no match for bedside discussions of side effects, drug-drug interactions, cost, and how many times a day the patient would have to remember to take a pill. It was not that the basic science wasn't important; it was just that a more immediate set of details, at a scale directly relevant to the patient, were now the trees we needed to see in order to make big-picture treatment decisions.

The second contrast was that medical research almost always involved large groups of people, but we have to make medical decisions on a case by case basis. However, studies with small groups, and especially sing-patient case reports, are generally looked upon with skepticism by the medical community. The rise of what became known as evidence-based medicine happened for a good reason: we cannot draw the best scientific conclusions from individual experiences, which are cluttered with details that may or may not apply to the next patient and are difficult to tease apart from a host of potential biases in decision-making and interpretations. This makes good sense in many ways. But these reasons we use to justify larger studies are often the very same reasons that we may not be able to apply these larger studies to individual patient decisions. Details that are important for an individual might get blurred by averaging over a large group, or the group might not have even included any people quite like the patient sitting in front of us. I learned more than just the need to see both the forest and the trees. Perhaps more importantly, I learned that knowing whether what we are looking at is the forest or the trees can be tricky and can be different in different situations.

Context is the key

The spirit of personalized medicine, or what is now more commonly called precision medicine, captures this tension between the forest and the trees. A more practical approach, which I try to keep in mind with each patient, is that for any aspect of health, we should be able to answer two questions: how worried should we be, and what options do we have if we are worried enough to act. It's a simple reminder that data becomes more powerful when we provide the context of a person's story, and a person's story becomes more actionable when we add the context of data. Among the possible actions we can take—including whether to act at all—the most sensible decisions arise when we remember the importance of context. Context offers some insulation against uncertainty when it arises, like when experts disagree or when research publications present unexpected findings. We make many decisions in life and in health with imperfect information, and decisions about sleep are no different. I wrote this book to confront some of the most common uncertainties head-on: not to vanquish them like mythical monsters but rather to wrap these thorny buggers in the gentle blanket of context.

My sleep story

Maybe the stage was set at an early age for me to eventually become a sleep special-ist. My father loves to tell this story, and it's one of the few stories from my child-hood for which I'm not embarrassed to remain in the room. I was a sleep-walker as a child—actually a "sleep-runner," as my parents recall—and this continued into my medical-school years, much to my roommates' chagrin. I was also quite the sleep-talker, and my sleep-talking persists to this day. My wife says it usually involves me sounding upset about some statistics topic, so in that way my sleep-talking seems pretty reflec-tive of my waking life. Anyway, one night when I was very young, maybe four years old, I walked downstairs, where my father was watching TV, and said, "Where is it?" over and over. My father was pretty comfortable on the couch, he recalls, and having noticed that I was actually asleep and that he'd have to carry me back up to my room, he cleverly said, "It's in your bed." And like magic, away I walked, right back upstairs. But before he could high-five my mother, apparently I'd wandered back downstairs, stood next to him, still asleep, and said, "It's not there." I like this story because of the combination of tacitly calling out my father on being too lazy to carry me up the first time and the fact that my disposition for arguing is so deep-seated that it persists even in sleep.

In addition to sleep-walking and sleep-talking, I've always been a night owl. I've been through every alarm, dawn simulator, and bedtime experimentation known to humanity. I'm not sure how I got through my residency training without ever being late to morning rounds on the patient wards. Some people outgrow this night-owl tendency over time, but for me it actually got worse after my residency—it was so bad that I wouldn't schedule meetings in the morning when I first began my faculty position at Massachusetts General Hospital. The only successful cure, for me, was to marry a morning person. At least I'm going to assume that was my cure, since I can't conduct a randomized trial to prove it.

The first night I spent in a sleep lab myself (to undergo a full clinical polysomnogram), I was in the midst of my junior-faculty night-owl career, and the lab had a last-minute cancellation—so I jumped at the chance. I had no idea how important that night would be for me as a sleep doctor. I had wanted to experience what patients felt like under the wraps of all of those sensors. I had also wanted to test out several wearable devices we were using for at-home sleep-tracking research. I was wrapped in the regular sleep-test sensors plus about eight other sleep monitoring devices. Although I rarely have trouble sleeping, it turned out on that night I found myself really struggling from the get-go. I could hear snoring in the next room through the wall. I could hear the technologist's voice talking to another patient over the intercom. The regular clinical sensors and extra devices made me more uncomfortable than I expected, as someone who regularly brags about being able to sleep in any setting. Part of me was even probably a little giddy with anticipation of getting some highly detailed personal sleep data for the first time. But here I was, in a pitch-black room, staring at the tiny red light glowing from the oxygen sensor and wondering what I had gotten myself into. While I usually measure my sleep onset time in seconds, on this night it felt like an eternity to fall asleep. Even after I finally dozed off, I woke up several times and had trouble falling back asleep.

Or so I thought.

In the morning, after the technologist helped to remove all the sensors and goop, I filled out the customary post-test questionnaire to give my subjective estimates of how the night had gone: the exact same questions we ask all our patients the morning after their sleep tests are completed:

Question 1: How long did it take you to fall asleep after lights out? My guess was: "Two hours." I've never taken that long to fall asleep, and recalling it the next morning made me cringe.

Question 2: If you woke up during the night, for how long? I was guessing again here, admittedly: "One hour," I estimated, from being awake three or four times, each of about fifteen minutes or so.

Question 3: How long do you think you slept, in total? This question gave me pause. It occurred to me that I usually know how long I've slept only from calculating the difference between my bedtime and my morning alarm. This night was different because I had a lot of awake time to account for. So I tried to go through the calculations. I was in bed for about 6.5 hours in total (11:30 p.m. was lights out, and at 6:00 a.m. the technologist came in to end the test). From 6.5 hours of time in bed, I subtracted two hours for my sleep-onset estimation, and subtracted one additional hour for my estimate of awake-time during the night. This left me with a total sleep duration estimate of just 3.5 hours.

And boy did I feel zonked out that next day. I went about my work day as best I could, with some extra coffee, of course. It wasn't until the following day that I was able to review my own sleep data from the testing night. Here I was, a board-certified sleep neurologist, directing funded research studies of sleep and perception, and I couldn't believe my own eyes. It hadn't taken me two hours to fall asleep—It hadn't even been twenty minutes! By two hours after lights out, which was my estimate of the delay to sleep onset, I had already cycled through deep slow-wave sleep, and my first block of REM sleep was just ending. I did subsequently awaken several times during the night, but each time was for under two minutes. It sure felt longer than that! The total sleep time was almost six hours, according to my EEG data. I was shocked, and I even felt a little embarrassed: What kind of a sleep neurologist can't tell if he's awake or asleep? I strained to re-create my memory of the night. The time when I'd felt awake was not unusual in any way: not foggy, not uncertain at all. The time when I'd felt awake was just like any other time I'd felt awake. I felt fully conscious, which was no different than my "regular" waking experience: thoughts, sounds, sensations, even looking at the clock. Not a clue could be found to hint that I'd been asleep or even in some kind of intermediate state between sleep and wake.

Ever since that night, every time I care for a patient with insomnia who experiences this disconnect of perception, I recall my own sensation of being awake that night as being as terrifically "real" as any other waking experience. When patients learn of that disconnect for themselves, they're often totally shocked to hear that they could have been asleep while feeling so awake, just like in my case. I can validate their feeling. I can relate to their experience as someone who's shared it, even if only on rare nights like that one in the lab.

The sleep medicine literature has long recognized sleep misperception. Until recently, researchers might have viewed sleep misperception as a scientific curiosity that raised questions about the nature of our conscious experience. But new data in the past five years (since 2012 or so) has shown that misperception has graduated from being a mere curiosity to having a seat at the table of real-world clinical decision-making.[a] And that's where the magic occurs for me. Sometimes academic physicians like me feel like we wear two hats—one in the research lab, and another in the clinic—and if we're lucky, the two worlds overlap from time to time. For any topic in sleep medicine, whether I'm listening to a research lecture, talking to a patient in the clinic, or performing my own research, I keep coming back to two basic questions: How worried should we be, and what can we do about it if we are worried enough to act? This is why I look at sleep medicine like an adventure, where context is the guiding principle that shapes decision-making—and context comes from your sleep story.

Where to next?

You don't need to be a full-time sleep geek to think of sleep as an adventure. Everyone's sleep story has twists and turns and parts that are more or less memorable. There may be conflict and (I hope) resolution in your adventure. You'll meet all sorts of characters along the way, and sometimes even sleep doctors will make appearances. You'll have choices and trade-offs to make using incomplete information. Now that you've been peppered with some uncertainty in this chapter, it's time to make a very practical decision: Where to next? Look over the table of contents, and if one of the chapter titles pops out as something that sounds interesting, then your adventure goes there next. If you're trembling with uncertainty at the risk-benefit balance of chapter choice, I can tip the balance on this one decision for you: turn the page to chapter 2.

---

a See chapter 17 for more on sleep perception.

CHAPTER 2
What's a sleep lab?

(I welcome a medical student to the lab to learn about sleep medicine[a])

et's start at the beginning. There's something exciting about showing people what sleep looks like. You can't predict their response. When the people you are showing something are medical students, their mixture of fear and excitement with new exposures is based more on book knowledge than personal experience. For patients, the mixture is more likely to be the opposite: heavily weighted by personal experience. Context shapes the way we receive and interpret information, especially if that information is unexpected or anxiety provoking, such as test results from a night in the sleep lab—which itself can be anxiety provoking! Several times a year, I welcome trainees and medical students to the sleep lab to learn about sleep medicine, and looking at overnight sleep data from our lab is an ideal starting point. After reading thousands of these reports, when I have the opportunity to teach students, I am reminded to pause and think about how it feels to sit for the first time in front of a geeky overload of physiologic signals cascading across a computer screen.

"Sometimes the patient falls asleep sitting in the chair while the technician is still applying the sensors—before the recording even starts. Here, luckily, we'll see the transition to sleep. The lights are turned off, but the night-vision camera shows the blaze of a smartphone and the sharp deflections of the sensors around the eyes as they dart through whatever the patient felt the need to read before bedtime."

---

a Think of this chapter as a conversation I'm having with a medical student rotating through my sleep clinic. The quotes are me speaking, and the headings are the student's questions.

Do we let patients use their phones in the lab after lights out?

Medical students (perhaps students in general) are a study in themselves, and their questions can be quite telling about an always-interesting topic: How is a field perceived by those outside the field? We haven't even begun our session, and I'm resisting what will seem at first like a tangent but over time will seem more central: that even common and simple-sounding ideas may not be so simple in sleep medicine.

"We'll come back to that question later, when we talk about a concept called ecological validity[b]. For now, the answer is that we want this night, for the most part, to reflect what home sleep would have been like. Patients are typically free to eat a snack, look at their phones, watch a bit of TV, bring in their special pillow, and take their usual nighttime medications."

What if light exposure or medications affect the testing results?

"Perfect questions—and it's at the heart of what we'll talk about over and over again in the sleep clinic: How do we balance theoretical and practical, risks and benefits, research world and real world? For the light question, surprising as it may sound, the sleep testing is not designed to test melatonin levels or light-related sleep disturbances.[c] For the medication question, many medications do affect sleep, but abruptly stopping them could also have an impact on sleep. In many cases, it's the problem with stopping a medication abruptly that is to be avoided. Think of a person who usually takes a nightly sleeping pill and then, because of concerns it might affect the results, stops it just for the night of testing in the sleep lab. Stopping abruptly could cause a kind of withdrawal insomnia, and getting less sleep in the lab means that we have less information from the test. This problem of symptoms resuming can happen when other medications are abruptly stopped as well, such as anxiety or pain or restlessness. Measuring patients as close to how they are sleeping at home—and that unfortunately includes nightly sleeping pills for some—allows us to make personalized recommendations from the results. Many patients, very reasonably, are interested in knowing if certain medications are affecting their sleep. And if those medications can be tapered safely, then this can be done in the weeks or months prior to the overnight test."

---

b See chapters 4 and 19 for more on the topic of validation.
c See chapter 18 for more details about sleep testing.

I had the feeling my student was only partially satisfied with my explanation. "There's one thing we do in the lab—besides apply all these sensors—that might be different than a typical night in the home: we want to make sure we catch the person sleeping supine—on his back, in this case—especially during a dream. When anyone hears this, patient or student (or another physician!), the immediate question arises: What if a person doesn't sleep on his back at home?

"A person's breathing during sleep may worsen while on his back. We'll talk more about snoring and sleep apnea,[d] which are the main reasons for visiting the overnight sleep lab. One of the most interesting and useful observations about sleep apnea is that it can change severity depending on someone's body position during sleep. For some people, we observe sleep apnea *only* when they're sleeping on their backs. That's why we want to make sure we see people in this vulnerable condition.

"This is another great example of needing to balance the real world and the medical world. If we could rely on a person's report of body position in sleep, then your instinct would be exactly right that we should not force her into that position in the testing lab. But in this case, it's not so easy, and getting this wrong can have important consequences. For many people, body position changes quite a bit throughout the night: a recent study showed in over six hundred adults that body-position changes occurred one to two times per hour, on average.[12] Since we are not aware of most of these shifts, it's not surprising that someone might not know how much time was spent sleeping in any particular position. We looked into this in a study[13] comparing the video data to the patient report of how much time people spent on their backs, and while some people were quite accurate, there was a large range of uncertainty. Since we can't predict which people are accurate (or not) in their awareness or recollections of body position while sleeping, we want to at least measure body position in the sleep lab, and how sleep apnea changes with body position, so that we'll know how worried we should be if people were to sleep on their backs in the home. This is equally important for sleep apnea treatment suggestions,[e] since the common advice to avoid sleeping on your back works best if we know you only have sleep apnea in that body position."

---

d See chapters 7 and 8 for more on sleep apnea.

e See chapter 11 for more on position therapy for sleep apnea.

MATT BIANCHI MD, PHD

How can people sleep with all this equipment?

"The lights have just been turned off. We can tell the patient is awake here, with his eyes blinking and darting back and forth, which we see as pointy rapid waveforms from the sensors next to his eyes. We click a few more screens forward—each screen is thirty seconds of time—and now we see what 'drowsy' looks like on our sensors: as his eyes close, the small irregular jitters of the EEG (electroencephalogram) we see while you're awake organize into a clearly different pattern of waves. This is the 'alpha' rhythm—the uncreative term for the first pattern ever seen by the doctor credited with the first EEG recordings almost a hundred years ago. As the story goes, Dr. Berger was intent to understand mental telepathy and psychic energy from the brain, but his contemporaries largely dismissed him for over a decade until people recognized his insights as a tool to study brain physiology with sensors attached to the scalp. Anyway, most people anticipate difficulty sleeping under the wraps of all these sensors, but the good news is we almost always get enough information to act on, even if it's not the ideal of comfort.

"Soon we see that the eye movements are now slow and rolling back and forth—and the EEG alpha pattern gives way to slower and more irregular waves. The breathing slows and becomes more regular, and with it the heartbeat slows down. If you squint a little, you can see that the breathing and the heart rate are connected: each exhale slows the heart rate down, and each inhale speeds it up again. See this squiggle in the vibration sensor? The snoring has already begun—one of the symptoms that we know from the intake forms prompted this patient to come to the sleep lab for testing. As we keep advancing the screens forward, we also see a series of leg twitches, each less than a second long; in this case, we can't even see them on the video but we pick them up with sensors on each leg. Most people with restless legs syndrome do have leg twitches while asleep, in addition to the uncomfortable sensations they feel while awake. But most people with leg twitches during sleep, which we call periodic limb movements, have no noticeable leg symptoms while they're awake. That's the case in this patient, whose only sleep complaint was snoring."[f]

How much information can we get in just one night?

The best learning opportunities start with questions rooted in skepticism. "You've really hit the nail on the head with that question. Especially when patients are getting

f See chapter 16 for more on restless legs syndrome and periodic limb movements of sleep.

unexpected results, this is a common first question: Was that night really representative? Most people have good intuition, from their personal experience, that sleep quality and quantity can be affected by many things that might change from day to day, like alcohol or caffeine or stress, but also by factors that might change over longer time scales, like medications or weight gain. With each of our patients, we must place the data we obtain from their sleep tests into the context of their stories. Most of my job is to help people navigate uncertainty, since we face so much of it. Most kinds of uncertainty we can deal with, but we also need to admit when we don't understand something well enough to have a clear answer. Sleep data only makes sense in the context provided by the patient's story. All patients make decisions or plans based on some combination of their story and their data."

Do some people really stop breathing when they sleep?

We click through another dozen screens, showing some snoring and a few leg twitches, and then we stop for a new pattern. "Here we can see that the breathing sensors have started to dwindle, with a slight reduction in heart rate as the breaths get smaller. Then, about twenty seconds later, we see that the breathing kicks back in, with even larger breaths than before. These are what we call recovery breaths, following the interruption, and we see the heart rate speed up a bit at that time."

The wide eyes remind me that I have to recalibrate myself for a moment. We see so many interruptions in breathing, far more disruptive than this example, such that we need to take a moment for context. "This is another key point. Sleep apnea is a common problem, and we use the data from tests like this to help figure out how worried we should be. The average duration of a breathing interruption is twenty to thirty seconds, but sometimes it can be sixty seconds or longer. Seeing someone stop breathing while sleeping can be a frightening prospect, even for ten seconds, especially if you happen to be the person's bed partner. If we place these interruptions in context, we'll see that the duration is not necessarily the main concern. The best data to tell us about the severity of sleep apnea is how frequently a person's breathing is interrupted during sleep, rather than the duration of each individual event. Actually, having some pauses in breathing is generally considered normal, and some people are surprised that, to make the diagnosis of sleep apnea, we need to observe at least five breathing interruptions *per hour of sleep*. We consider that amount of breathing interruption, and up to as high as fifteen interruptions per hour, to be a mild case of sleep apnea."

Aren't certain sleep stages more important than others?

"Let's zoom ahead to look at rapid eye movement, or REM, sleep, but we'll pause first on some non-REM sleep for comparison. We're now in the midst of a long bout of non-REM stage 2, or N2 for short. This is where we see waveforms called spindles and K-complexes, and tons of research has gone into determining what these might mean for our understanding of brain function during sleep. But this research has not yet reached the point of real-world decision-making, which is our focus in the clinic. As an aside, N2 comprises most of what most of the consumer sleep monitoring devices call 'light sleep,' a curious name that incorrectly makes it sound unimportant.

"I'm probably starting to sound like a broken record: this is another aspect of sleep medicine that has a surprising gap between the research world and the real world. We can definitely see different sleep problems in REM versus non-REM stages, so in that sense, the sleep stages are important for some diagnoses. But we don't have good evidence to show that directly changing the amount of a given stage is important for health, not to mention that we have no clinical tools to increase these stages.[g] One common issue is that most sleeping pills, if they increase sleep duration at all, do so by increasing time spent in stage N2. Most sleeping pills and many of the other medications used in neurology and psychiatry reduce the amount of REM sleep we get. I'm not convinced that we understand these observations well enough to affect our clinical decision-making. I'm more concerned about certain medications worsening breathing during sleep, or worsening the leg twitches during sleep.

"Just ahead we can see a big change: the EEG looks irregular again, and the eyes are darting back and forth quickly—very similar to the beginning of the night, when the patient was awake and looking at his phone. But in the video feed, we can see the lights are out, and there is no phone in sight. Do these rapid eye movements mean the patient has woken up?"

The slight smirk from the student as I draw out the phrase *rapid eye movements* in my question lets me know the point is understood: here the rapid eye movements are not from being awake, but rather from entering REM sleep. "Another clue that this person is asleep rather than awake is that we still hear snoring. So here we are seeing the famously storied REM stage of sleep. I can even tell what this patient is dreaming about."

The smirk is replaced by raised eyebrows this time. Too dry a joke for the student's first day on the sleep medicine elective rotation. "I'm kidding, of course, and

---

g See chapter 18 for more on sleep stages.

that's a good thing for all parties involved. Anyway, REM sleep was first discovered and named by sleep researchers in the early 1950s, more than twenty years after the first EEG recordings of sleep were made. It turned out that much of what you could measure about REM sleep looked just like the awake state: irregular breathing, variable heart rate, rapid eye movements, and even the EEG squiggles. This data was so striking that much of the early literature referred to REM as 'paradoxical sleep,' because it looked so much like being awake. In the original 1953 publication describing REM sleep,[14] the researchers observed this distinct phase of sleep by noting three distinct features compared to the rest of the night: rapid eye movements, wake-like EEG squiggles, and irregular breathing patterns. So we now uncreatively call this phase of sleep REM—but it could easily be called 'irregular respiration sleep,' although that doesn't exactly roll off the tongue. Even this 1953 description was not the first to notice that breathing patterns changed during sleep. I stumbled upon a book from 1891, *Insomnia and Its Therapeutics*,[15] which opens by commenting that careful observation of respirations shows that, occasionally in the night, the breathing pattern would wax and wane, which the author dismisses as an observation 'without any special significance,' in his opinion."

We scroll through the patient's recording for another hour, looking at examples of different sleep stages, brief awakenings, different muscle twitches, and even some pauses in breathing. "Let's step back now to summarize all these squiggles over the seven hours of sleep for the clinical report: we counted twenty-eight breathing interruptions, sixty-eight leg twitches, and fifty-one brief arousals from sleep. I'll provide a written interpretation of this study as demonstrating snoring but otherwise normal sleep findings."

I don't usually need to draw out the word *normal* for students to seem surprised, as if maybe they'd heard me wrong. "Yes, normal sleep can look quite bumpy when we actually record it objectively with sensors. How bumpy, and in what ways, helps us decide how worried we should be and what treatment options are available. In this case, I remember from the prior clinic visit that this patient wasn't aware of his own snoring, and it was his family members who were both bothered and concerned. After this particular testing night in the lab, when we asked the patient in the morning to reflect back on the night, he thought he'd only been asleep for four hours, but the EEG showed that he'd been asleep for six and a half hours. We've already talked about how our awareness of body position, snoring, and leg twitches may or may not match up with our perceptions or symptoms. It turns out that even our feelings of being asleep versus awake might not match up.[h] These aren't just curiosities; they are recognized points of uncertainty that can affect how we make decisions, and being aware of them is an important step when we think of placing information in context for each patient."

h See chapter 17 for more about perceptions of sleep.

CHAPTER 3

How much sleep should I get?

Would that this were a simple question

You might expect this to be a very short chapter. We even have an official answer to the title's question: in 2015 the American Academy of Sleep Medicine published its recommendations on this topic.[6] For healthy adults, the recommendation is that we get seven hours or more sleep per night. We could reinforce this seemingly simple recommendation by referencing key research findings about the importance of sleep for our health and well-being. While I admit that "Insufficient sleep is bad for you" could be the least controversial headline of all time, I nevertheless find myself struggling with this common question of how much sleep a person should get. Perhaps it's because when people ask me this question, they are thinking of their own sleep, and so the question is not "How much does the average person need?" but rather "How much sleep do *I* need, Doctor?" This is a common theme in medicine, though it is not always easy to address: how to apply knowledge derived from studying groups of people to decisions and actions for an individual. So, this question gets more than a short chapter.

Let's explore whether the question of "How much sleep do you need?" is as easy as it sounds, like it should be. What if it's like asking how much food should you eat? For that question, we can look to average daily recommendations: about two thousand calories for women, and about twenty-five hundred for adult men. Of course, there are many exceptions, depending on your health status, weight goals, exercise habits, and so on. It is not surprising to think that we may or may not want to apply the average suggestion to individuals without taking into account their specific contexts. We can take this analogy a bit further. Food isn't one thing (fortunately!), and the total amount of calories we consume in an average day might not seem to be the most sensible way to capture the role of food in our health. Likewise, the duration of sleep is just one way to think about sleep, and a person who's thinking about sleep for health or performance reasons might also want to think about the timing and quality of sleep.

It's probably not too much of a stretch to think that it might be useful to consider sleep quality as well as quantity. Is this just some Socratic exercise, like saying, "Sure, Doctor, you might recommend eight glasses of water per day, but what if the water's contaminated with cholera?" If that's your instinct—perfect! We want to maintain a healthy balance of skepticism: that's part of the adventure—figuring out what is most relevant and applicable to your context. So yes, cholera-contaminated water is bad, but if you have the luxury of clean water, then we can get back feeling comfortable talking about the eight glasses of water recommendation. Oh, that is, unless you are experiencing heart failure. Or if you've just run a marathon. Or if your sodium level in the blood is low. The point is, there are always what ifs, but only some of those ifs will be relevant for a specific person.

Some authorities suggest that we can answer the question of how much sleep do you need by seeing what happens when you don't set an alarm. That might seem clever or at least harmless enough to think that our brains know to wake up naturally after being satisfied we've had the right amount of sleep. Let's play out this idea and think about what happens if you pick a day and don't set an alarm; whenever you wake up, that's how you will know when you've had enough sleep. If we unpack the thinking of this experiment, we don't have to dig too deeply to realize that this isn't such a simple experiment after all. What if you wake up after three hours of sleep—maybe to use the bathroom, or for no apparent reason? Does it mean your body is done for the night, or just done for the time being? Does that answer depend on whether you're able to fall back asleep quickly? What if you do the no-alarm experiment several days in a row, and the total duration of sleep is a range from five to ten hours from night to night: Which is the "right" one? Does the answer to that question depend on how you feel upon waking? And if you really carried out such an experiment,[a] tracking how many hours you sleep without an alarm and tracking how refreshed you feel each day, wouldn't you also need to keep track of (or eliminate) any other factors that might affect your quality or quantity of sleep, or how much energy you have while awake, so that you could actually interpret the results of this sleep-without-an-alarm experiment?

---

a See chapter 19 for more on self-discovery.

An interlude about food

If we think back to the food analogy, we'd expect that many factors would play a role in deciding how much you would eat when unrestricted (such as at a buffet), only one of which is your biological caloric need. How palatable is the food, how much have you eaten recently, what are your exercise patterns and metabolism like, and do you know when your next meal will be—each of these could affect buffet consumption. Our sense of hunger depends on many factors, and so hunger may or may not reflect our biological need for more calories. When we overeat, even if it feels good to do so, we should not assume that this consumption is rooted in a biological need for those extra calories. Clearly, many factors are involved in our food intake beyond biological caloric need. Similarly, for sleep, how much you have slept (or not slept) recently, as well as the timing and quality of that sleep, are some of the factors that might come into play when you sleep without an alarm.

Taking the analogy further, research is showing that calorie restriction and even intermittent fasting may actually be good for our health in some situations. Although it may be hard to imagine a parallel with sleep restriction, we actually don't have to dig too deeply to find one. It turns out that acute sleep deprivation, usually meaning lack of sleep for one night, can be euphoric and has been extensively studied as a therapy for depression—an entire chapter of my sleep textbook *Sleep Deprivation* was dedicated to this technique[16]. While this is obviously a niche topic and is not widely implemented in clinical practice, the point is that we can hardly find an aspect of sleep that isn't more complicated—and interesting—than we might have thought. The book you're reading now is about not shying away from uncertainty and gray areas, but rather thinking through how sleep information plays a role (or not) in your particular context.

Sleep duration: a new take on Goldilocks

What if you are one of the many people who find that they feel worse if they sleep for too long—should you follow your body's "natural" idea (which you discovered from not setting an alarm) and allow the extended sleep duration, even at the cost of feeling worse upon waking? Would it be like forcing yourself to eat spinach, even though it doesn't appeal to you—or even causes, say, nausea—because it's supposed to be healthy? Some people have a range that seems to feel best to them, and they find themselves non-refreshed when they get less or more than this "sweet spot." Others feel the same energy no matter how much they sleep, unless the duration is very short. We haven't even scratched the surface of the different ways to measure sleep *quality*, and we see that even asking questions about sleep *quantity* is not always straightforward.

Before we think about trying the no-alarm experiment, we might want to first think about whether we are the kind of person for whom such an experiment would make sense. I would need to be a person who wakes up with an alarm regularly (so I can try not setting the alarm), whose sleep quality is normal (so I can focus on sleep duration), who is willing to not set an alarm for at least a week (to get a decent average), and who is willing to track or control other factors that can influence the relationship between sleep duration and daytime energy (like naps, caffeine, alcohol, and exercise).

The problem of thinking about the brain knowing when to wake us up is even more complicated when we consider that the sleeping brain is actually "waking up" many times during a normal night of sleep, whether we realize it or not. How many times? You guessed it—it depends. If we only count the awakenings we are consciously aware of, then the average person might have none, or a couple, in a given night. If we count awakenings according to the clinical scoring rules during a sleep lab test (which is at least fifteen seconds long on the sleep EEG sensors), then these kinds of awakenings may happen a dozen times in a single night of sleep. If we count shorter awakenings between three and fifteen seconds long (called "arousals" in the clinical scoring rules), then we can see a dozen of these *per hour of sleep* in the average normal adult!

Maybe it's not so surprising after all that the approach of "my body will let me know" isn't so simple. Thinking about other aspects of our daily lives, it seems the way our bodies tell us things is more like poetry than like a user manual. Does my body tell me to stop eating only when I've met my caloric needs for the day? How much water do I need to drink today? Was this exercise session I've just done the right intensity? We might have clues about these kinds of things that might be more or less vague or intense, depending on the person and the situation. It seems like we could more strongly argue that none of the body's systems are designed to be exquisitely tuned. Rather, just about everything we know about human biology suggests that the situation is quite the opposite: for healthy adults, our body systems are equipped to maintain function in the face of unpredictable and fluctuating environments. Of course, in certain diseases, this resilience or adaptability can be compromised, and even basics like water intake can tip a system out of balance. Our body systems are affected by age, genetics, medications, health problems, and even recent exposures and experiences. Sleep is no different. Thinking about sleep duration requires the context provided by health status, recent sleep history, waking needs, and availability of countermeasures to compensate for deficits in performance or function while awake. Even the performance question can be personalized: experiencing drowsiness behind a desk carries different risks than drowsiness behind the wheel of a vehicle.

One more example is worth mentioning, which relates to the often-asked question of paying back sleep debt. In other words, can a person catch up on lost sleep, say, on weekends? A certain kind of research experiment is often cited to answer this with a "No, you can't completely catch up on sleep debt." The experiments usually involve keeping people up all night, and then the following night allowing them to sleep as much as they wish. It turns out that the sleep duration on the recovery night is not double the normal duration, to make up for the zero sleep on the prior night. Instead, recovery sleep after a night of total deprivation is typically about 1.5 times the typical sleep duration. The "no" interpretation to catch-up sleep is based on this failure to add back the whole prior night's worth of missing sleep time. Another interpretation of this observation is that you pay off sleep debt at a discount of sorts: that you don't need all that sleep time to catch up, from a biological standpoint, at least for short-term sleep loss. One of the legends in sleep research, Dr. Jim Horne, has written about this concept of core sleep versus optional sleep, which might play into the discounted payback interpretation. The fact that catch-up sleep does not represent one-to-one payback should also give us pause about the suggestion that the right amount of sleep to get is "whenever you wake up without an alarm." If the brain knows best, then the partial payback of sleep debt is in fact biologically appropriate.

Let's get back to the official medical recommendation for adults to get seven hours or more of sleep. The American Academy of Sleep Medicine performed a rigorous review of the literature, described in a twenty-three-page methodological publication[17] accompanying the brief two-page summary recommendation.[6] Some might find it surprising to hear that the academy's conclusions were what we call in the medical world "consensus," which is the lowest rung on the evidence ladder. This means the research evidence was low quality, but experts agreed on a recommendation based on experience and what information was available. Can this question of sleep duration really be so difficult to answer? Surely the canon of biomedical research can claim this knowledge somewhere amid its spoils? We've already discussed some of the challenges, but see what you think as we peek behind the evidence curtain.

The academy report was careful to emphasize that the recommendations were for healthy adults. It also highlighted three particular weak spots in the available research it drew from. First, nearly all the research into sleep duration was based on asking people how much they slept on average—a subjective rather than objective assessment. Second, while many studies reported a correlation between sleep duration and various health risks, none could prove that sleep duration *caused* the risk. Third, even the correlations turned out to be a little strange: in addition to shorter sleep durations correlating with a variety of bad health outcomes, longer-than-average sleep durations were even worse for health! Many experts have weighed in on this U-shaped risk pattern,[18-21] referring to the shape of a graph where average sleep duration—usually seven hours—has the lowest health risk, and increased risk occurs for both lower and higher sleep durations.

We can make the point about correlation versus causation a little more concrete: none of the research answered the key question an individual would want to know: will changing our habitual sleep duration improve or reverse any of the health risks that correlated with short (or long!) sleep duration? In other words, if you typically get six hours of sleep per night, whether you feel good or bad about that amount subjectively, there is little evidence that increasing your sleep duration to seven or eight hours will improve your health. (To make things even more complicated, other research has shown that using medications to extend sleep is linked to the same kinds of problems as the short-duration sleep![b]) For such a fundamental question of the health benefits of sleep extension, only a handful of limited studies have been published.[22-25] Likewise, no evidence exists for any benefits if you're a ten-hours-per-night kind of person who's deprived yourself of sleep down to eight hours. For a final touch of skepticism of self-reported sleep duration (as opposed to measuring sleep objectively), we need look no further than studies showing that the answers given to "How much sleep did you get?" depend on who you ask, when you ask, and how you ask.[26-28] This should at least give us pause when we interpret research studies based on self-reported sleep duration, especially if they are making health-related claims from the results.

How can both shorter and longer than average sleep duration be linked to health risks? Is the Goldilocks fable relevant for sleep health? The most common explanation is that while the short sleep durations cause health problems, the long sleep durations are *caused by* health problems. In other words, the argument is that the U-shaped correlations of health risk and sleep duration only have causality on one side (the short duration side). That could be true. But each research study reporting U-shaped risk correlations did their best to account for other health problems across all sleep durations, not just one side of the average. We'd have to suppose that some hidden

---

b See chapter 13 for more on sleeping pills.

health problems were uniquely present in the long sleepers to make them sleep longer. Maybe we just can't imagine asking people to sleep *less* to improve their health! This problem of correlating sleep duration with health is a nice example of needing to place data in context: data does not, as the saying goes, speak for itself. For anyone who's already shuddering at the statistical terms of correlation and causation, consider visiting Harvard Law School graduate Tyler Vigen's website (www.tylervigen.com/spurious-correlations) for countless examples of accidental correlations to get the big picture here: it's one thing to find a *correlation* in data, but if we're going to take action, then we need to dig deeper and think about the possibility of *causation*.

Is there a downside to recommendations on healthy sleep duration?

Some people might find all this nit picking about research studies simply a distraction from what should be common sense. Maybe it feels like the greater goal here is addressing the epidemic sleep loss of modern high-tech, high-stress society, and that getting buried in the uncertainties of research might derail that goal. To that sentiment, I would feel like agreeing, but even this idea of a modern epidemic of sleep loss seems to be overstated. One of the most powerful arguments against this idea was a detailed 2016 analysis of over 150 prior research studies conducted over the past half century, which concluded that no change in sleep duration or quality had occurred over this time frame.[7,29] The aforementioned Dr. Horne spent much of his 2016 book *Sleeplessness* poring over the available research to arrive at the same conclusion.[30] Another legend in the sleep field, Dr. Jerome Siegel, has studied sleep in preindustrial societies using objective monitoring; he found that sleep durations tended to be *lower* in such societies than among adults who live in modern communities.[31] Some people might still feel like these disagreements should live comfortably tucked away in academic ivory towers, and we should instead stick to common sense and get back to real-world recommendations. Since we're always reminding ourselves to consider the risk-benefit context, let's apply the same standard here: What are the downsides to recommending seven or more hours of sleep, given that the medical field offers similar-sounding general recommendations for health, like how much to exercise, how much water to drink, and how many servings of vegetables to eat per day?

I can think of the potential risks of sleep-duration recommendations for three kinds of people. One group consists of adults who sleep seven to eight hours per night already. They might be falsely reassured that their sleep is fine because of an over-focus on the single aspect of duration, and thus not take the next step of considering sleep quality.[c] Another group consists of adults with insomnia who are already concerned about the health implications of their problems with sleep and might mistakenly consider the recommended duration as a treatment goal.[d] To provide an idea of just how common this belief is, the first item on a validated questionnaire used in the insomnia field called "Dysfunctional Beliefs about Sleep" is "I need 8 hours of sleep." The third group consists of those who are healthy and feel fine but have always been relatively short sleepers and who might now think they have a sleep disorder simply because they are not meeting the recommended hours.

Who is most likely to benefit from healthy sleep duration recommendations?

We can table the research debates for a moment and take a more positive angle to consider who is most likely to benefit from a health recommendation of at least seven hours of sleep. One target audience immediately comes to mind: people who are taking sleep for granted and sacrificing the quantity they get, perhaps due to obligations of work or personal life. People who willingly forego some portion of their sleep may not appreciate the potentially detrimental effects that doing so has on their health. They may compensate for effects on performance with caffeine or power naps. By-choice sleep loss is different from medical problems that interfere with sleep, in that they can be resolved (at least in principle) by providing the opportunity to extend sleep. These people might reconsider the risk-benefit balance of their choices and strive to meet the recommended average.

If this is our main target audience, we can then ask: What portion of by-choice short sleepers will hear the academy's sleep recommendations and make choices that prioritize sleep and extend their sleep duration to at least seven hours? If we look by analogy at the history of recommending five daily servings of fruits and vegetables, public-service campaigns in the United States only slightly improved consumption,[32] and presumably that behavioral change would be easier than getting more sleep for many people. It turns out that trying to move beyond general recommendations to engage people with more active behavioral interventions to improve their health has only a modest and largely temporary impact.[33] But taking a page from our prior

---

c See chapter 5 for ways in which sleep quality can be poor even if you feel fine.
d See chapters 12 and 13 for more in insomnia.

argument that "the population might not apply to the individual," it seems likely that different people are motivated or inspired by different incentives. Context always matters. If temptation ever makes you think otherwise, then please reread the previous sentence. (Go ahead and do that now, just to be safe.)

Should we just say "we don't know" to the question of how much sleep should we get? We certainly don't want these challenges and uncertainties to open a path toward cavalier disregard for sleep. But with reputable voices in the sleep field coming to opposite conclusions about modern sleep patterns and the role of sleep duration in health, is this yet another tired case of "more research is needed"? Possibly, though unlike many other aspects of health, we can't perform the gold-standard clinical experiment, known as a randomized trial,[e] of sleep duration. Who would agree to enroll in a study to be randomly assigned to sleep short, long, or average durations every night for many years? Should we just throw our hands up at the uncertainty? Or is the conclusion that we should focus on developing ways for people to answer for themselves the questions of how worried they should be, and if they're worried enough to take action, how do they weigh their options? That's the theme we'll keep revisiting in this book (and we'll explore more about self-discovery, in particular, in chapter 19).

---

e See chapter 19 for more on randomized trials.

CHAPTER 4

My sleep tracker tells me...

Are consumer sleep-tracking devices accurate?

'm sure I sound like a broken record by now with always qualifying my answers, but here we go again: it depends. It's not like asking if your scale is an accurate measure of your weight. In that case, there is no claim or expectation of whether your weight is healthy or not, and if we don't trust the scale, it would not be hard to compare our weight using another device or gold standard, such as at a clinic. Sleep has many facets beyond duration, even in healthy people with no sleep problems. A fairer question for a sleep-tracking device would be to ask if it is accurate for a particular goal or category of information, and within each of those we can think through the uncertainties and how to address them.

Let's talk through the steps of what has to happen to interpret a sleep-monitoring device. First, the device's sensors have to measure something about you that we think is reliably linked to your sleep. Second, algorithms need to turn that sensor data into a prediction or score, such as being asleep versus awake or being in REM versus non-REM sleep. Neither of these steps is likely to be perfect, and the performance of each could very well change from person to person.

Let's talk about a few examples. In the old days, which in the sleep field means about 20 years ago, we used something called "actigraphy sensors" worn on the wrist, basically to measure movement. If you wore the device for several days in a row, we could look at the movement patterns and guess when you were awake or asleep. But years of research have shown—and you won't be surprised to hear this—that wrist movement is not always a great way of detecting whether a person is asleep or awake. For healthy adults, these motion trackers tend to overestimate sleep duration because even resting quietly could look like sleep if there was no movement happening. For people with certain sleep problems, movements might occur during sleep, creating the opposite kind of confusion for a motion sensor. In the sleep medicine field, we're now careful to call these devices "rest-activity" trackers, not "sleep-wake" trackers, to recognize this distinction and to avoid over-interpreting the information they provide.

Another example of tracker accuracy came from our experience with the Zeo sleep monitor, which was a headband that measured brain waves through forehead sensors. It was among the first consumer trackers to move beyond wrist tracking and report REM and non-REM components of sleep. Because of the position of the head-band, the sensors also picked up eye movements. As the name implies, we expect rapid eye movements during REM sleep. We also know, however, that certain medi-cations like antidepressants can increase eye movements during non-REM sleep so that these movements look similar to what we expect in REM. That's an example of how a medication might alter an algorithm's interpretation of data from a tracking sensor. We could also consider other reasons for algorithm performance issues, such as whether a person's sweat or the makeup someone wears might alter the headband sensor data. We commonly observe these kinds of sensor interference in other set-tings, like sweat affecting the EEG during an in-lab sleep test (polysomnogram), or when nail polish interferes with the oxygen sensors we often use on the fingertip to detect how well-oxygenated your blood is. Anyway, the makers of Zeo went out of business a few years ago, but several new headband-type EEG sensors are now (as of 2018) coming out in the consumer market. Time will tell how this new generation of technology will fare in terms of data quality at the sensor step and sleep tracking accuracy at the algorithm step.

It seems like it would be more useful to measure the stages, not just duration, of sleep

That's the million-dollar question! There is certainly a rich literature that has inves-tigated the role of REM and non-REM sleep in different kinds of memory and other restorative aspects of sleep. And it's not uncommon for patients in a clinic to ask about getting more REM sleep or more deep sleep. But these ideas and discoveries from the research world have not yet enjoyed practical application in the real world. It might come as a surprise to learn that the composition of sleep stages does not com-monly enter into clinical decision-making. Perhaps even more striking is the observa-tion that most medications used in neurology and psychiatry alter sleep stages, with the most common changes being *reduction*s in the amount of REM sleep or deep non-REM sleep. When people first started looking into medication effects several decades ago, one idea was that antidepressants worked to increase mood specifically because they suppressed REM sleep.[34,35] Although more recent work has not confirmed this idea,[36] there does not seem to be any adverse effect of altering sleep stages either. The take-home lesson for me is that if sleep stages can be affected by many factors—including many medications that suppress REM and deep sleep—then it's unclear how to reconcile that with the idea that memory and other cognitive processes are exquisitely tuned to sleep stages. Recent work has suggested that under more real-world conditions, there is little relationship between sleep-stage content and memory, for example.[37] This doesn't mean that we should simply disregard the research linking sleep stages to brain function or other aspects of health. Rather, it means that we should recognize that the relationships may be variable and difficult to act upon for any given individual.

The most curious part of this area for me is how this notion fits into treatment decisions. If someone really thinks REM is important for her functionality, would the possibility of suppressing REM figure into her decision to take an antidepressant or sleeping pill that could reduce her REM sleep? If we have any hope of helping people navigate these muddy waters, it could be through at-home sleep trackers. If we can overcome the limitations of accuracy, especially if the medications of interest themselves directly affect the tracker accuracy, the answer to how sleep stages affect our daily lives (or not) can be obtained on a case by case basis.

What does it mean for a consumer sleep tracking device to be "validated"?

In a perfect world, there would be no accuracy distinction between a consumer device you can buy without a doctor's order, and a medical-grade device used in clinical practice. In other aspects of health, people can buy something over the counter to measure themselves, like a scale or a thermometer, which in principle provides the same or similar information to what the doctor's office would obtain. Even blood pressure cuffs are routinely available for purchase, and the typical recommendation is to bring the device to the doctor to have it checked for accuracy and to make sure it's being used properly. These avenues of potentially frequent measurement in the home become extensions of what is measured during clinic visits that happen less frequently. There is growing interest in using such at-home information to improve healthcare in general, which could be conveyed to health-care providers between visits and provide greater real-world context to the data. With sleep trackers, it is perhaps less straightforward than that. It is not so easy to check the accuracy of a sleep tracker during a routine visit to the doctor, like you could with a blood pressure cuff.

I field the question "Which sleep trackers have been validated?" quite frequently, since this has been the focus of much of my research. The answer depends on a missing but necessary piece of the question: "For what?" Trackers measure different things about our physiology, and different algorithms turn those physiological measurements into outputs such as sleep-wake labels or sleep quality scores. This brings us to the two basic steps of tracking device validation. The first step is to show that a device's sensors reliably measure the physiology it claims to measure. How reliable is "reliable"? Well, that depends on the target audience. If you're tracking vital signs in an athlete during training, then you want your sensor to withstand motion and sweat, for example. With sleep, we might consider whether the device's sensors are affected by the presence of a bed partner, or by the type of bed you have, or by the temperature of the bedroom. We might consider the extent to which user error or variation in application details could affect the sensor, such as how tightly the device is worn or whether the position of the sensor on the body changes from night to night. For a device that's used on or near the bed, we might consider how changes in body position during the night could affect the sensor readings.

The second step is to show that the algorithms used to interpret the sensor data are accurate in whatever they claim to be reporting. For consumer devices, this typically means assigning a label of sleep versus wake, or of sleep stages like REM and non-REM, to the sensor data. Sometimes algorithms are created using data obtained from healthy young adults. But what if certain medical problems or sleep disorders confuse the accuracy of such an algorithm? Let's make this more concrete: say you have a tracker that measures breathing patterns, and it applies an algorithm to make predictions about REM versus non-REM stages throughout the night. Let's assume the sensor itself works perfectly to measure breathing, and also assume that in a healthy young adult, the algorithm perfectly predicts REM and non-REM sleep based on the person's breathing patterns. Now, what happens when a person with a breathing problem like sleep apnea uses the tracker? The device still measures breathing and still outputs a sequence of REM and non-REM stages, but how accurate is it, since sleep apnea directly alters the breathing-signal patterns? If the device were developed only on healthy adults without sleep apnea, the accuracy of sleep stages in someone with sleep apnea would likely be compromised, but we would not necessarily know that from the sequence of REM and non-REM outputs. Even if the device's algorithms were trained using examples of adults with sleep apnea, we could still ask the reasonable question: If someone has sleep apnea, should he be focusing on his sleep stages or should he make the breathing problem the first priority? (You can guess what my answer is likely to be!)

These topics are known in the research world as different forms of validation.[38] "Sensor validation" refers to the technical quality of the signal that's being measured. "Algorithm validation" usually begins with healthy adults who are studied in a controlled environment (like a sleep laboratory) against a gold standard such as polysomnography. The question of whether the algorithm would hold up if applied to a different population is called "external validity." The question of whether the device performance would hold up when used in the real world is called "ecological validity." This is why validation questions need to specify "for what" purpose.[a]

Can sleep trackers help raise awareness, even if the devices aren't accurate?

Now we're getting into the thick of it! So, the question is, could having inaccurate information be better than having no information if we attach a potential benefit like "increased awareness of the importance of sleep in general," which could simply mean not taking sleep for granted? I see the point, and phrased that way, I'd be inclined to agree that raising awareness is hard to argue with, so long as we aren't raising the awareness to anxiety levels. We discussed a similar "risk" question in chapter 3 regarding sleep duration. Let's say that a consumer sleep tracker only says that sleep is of "good" or "bad" quality, and the person who's using it feels her own experience as either "good" or "bad." These two views of sleep can be combined in four ways. But what about a gold-standard to know the true clinical status? For this, we'll also consider a third category—objective sleep according to clinical polysomnography testing in a sleep lab. Like the other categories, we will assume this test simply reports whether sleep quality was "good" or "bad". Now these, of course, are oversimplified, but let's see where it leads us. Eight possible combinations of these categories of information could happen. Let's map out the possibilities one by one. In each case, remember that most people don't have the luxury of the gold-standard polysomnogram test of a sleep lab—they're interpreting just two of the three categories of information (the tracker result and their own experience).

---

a See chapter 19 for more on the topic of validation.

Example #1: Feel good + tracker good + polysomnogram good
= Hooray! This situation is good. In this case, the tracker has provided accurate information relative to the gold-standard sleep test, which confirmed the subjective good feeling about sleep.

Example #2: Feel good + tracker good + polysomnogram bad
= Mistaken reassurance—the tracker did not detect a true problem that was visible on the polysomnogram. We can consider the tracker result to be a "false negative," because it failed to identify the truly bad sleep. Since the person felt good subjectively, he might not look any further to distinguish this scenario from example #1.

Example #3: Feel good + tracker bad + polysomnogram good
= Worried for no reason! This situation is not good. The tracker result is basically a "false positive," since it says that a sleep problem exists when none is present, by either gold-standard testing or by subjective feel. Here we run the risk of raising anxiety levels.

Example #4: Feel good + tracker bad + polysomnogram bad
= Tracker alerts the user to a sleep problem! Here, the tracker has correctly identified a sleep problem. The person feels fine, however, so she might distrust the tracker if she places more weight on her own experience.[b] She would need to obtain a polysomnogram to know whether she should trust the tracker or trust her subjective experience.

Example #5: Feel bad + tracker good + polysomnogram good
= The tracker is accurate but seems wrong. We have another disconnect here, as the person feels that his sleep is bad, but the tracker reports his sleep as good. Like example #4, he might not trust the tracker, but in this case, because of subjective symptoms, he might seek further testing with a polysomnogram.

---

b See chapter 8 for a common example of a sleep disorder that may not cause symptoms: sleep apnea.

Example #6: Feel bad + tracker good + polysomnogram bad

− The tracker provides false reassurance. Here, because the tracker has missed a true problem, we consider it a false negative result, like example #2. In this case, if the person trusts her experience over the tracker, she might pursue further testing with a polysomnogram. But what if she mistakenly accepts the reassurance from the tracker, perhaps because the trackers are marketed with language that makes them seem highly accurate?[38] That's a missed opportunity to seek help.

Example #7: Feel bad + tracker bad + polysomnogram good

= Tracker agrees with the subjective experience. This is a strange situation: the tracker seems to be capturing something that gold-standard testing doesn't see. Unless the tracker were so sophisticated that it could exceed modern diagnostics, which seems unlikely, we'd probably consider this case a false positive. But we wouldn't know for sure without the polysomnogram.

Example #8: feel bad + tracker bad + polysomnogram bad

= Believe it or not, this situation is actually good. In this case, we can consider the tracker result to be a "true positive" relative to the gold-standard poly-somnogram, having identified a sleep problem.

Examples #1 and #8 are the only two in which all three categories of information agreed. If we remember that most people don't have a polysomnogram to confirm their sleep status objectively (so they only consider the subjective feel and the tracker results), then we'll see that making decisions based on consumer trackers may not be as straightforward as we'd like. Chapters 8 and 17 dive into common situations in which how our sleep feels turns out to be different from what the sleep measurements reveal.

We arrived at this array of eight possibilities even after making a few simplifying assumptions, that sleep was either good or bad in each category. If we think beyond sleep being just good versus bad and start to consider other factors and sources of uncertainty in our own experience and in the data we get from devices, then it won't be surprising to learn that things get muddy in the real world where sleep quality exists on a spectrum. Although consumer trackers are not diagnostic devices, and doctors don't use them clinically to decide who needs a polysomnogram, we can see the potential for confusion, because the idea of sleep quality spans the wellness space of consumers and the medical space of clinics. When a well-meaning physician is quoted in a news story about consumer trackers as saying that such devices are fine for those who are curious, but those who have strong concerns about their sleep should talk to their doctors—this seems like a reasonably cautious stance. But the question remains, how should people figure out how worried they should be? Maybe when someone has clear sleep symptoms, or his family says he seems to struggle to breathe while he's asleep, these clues will raise concerns enough to motivate a medical evaluation. But what about those who have less clear symptoms, or even those who feel fine? How worried should they be, and could they be at risk for, say, sleep apnea?[c]

Imagine a man whose family tells him that he snores, and they're growing concerned about his sleep quality. He feels fine and isn't interested in bothering his doctor. In his defense, he pulls out his tracker, which gives him a high sleep-quality score. "You see? No problem," he says. What if the conversation stops there? What if the family counters that the tracker isn't designed to pick up snoring, so the next step is a snoring app? This might seem innocent enough. After a quick search of the various apps available, he does some monitoring and reluctantly admits that he snores. Let's say he then uses some home remedies for snoring, including applying breathing strips across the bridge of the nose, and his app says his snoring has improved. Case closed? Maybe—but without some medical-grade testing, we won't really know if he is "just" a snorer, or if he had sleep apnea, or, if he did have sleep apnea, how severe was it? Since snoring is not perfectly linked to sleep apnea, even if we believe the app is accurate and that his snoring has improved, it's possible that an underlying sleep-apnea problem remains. The issue, of course, is that you don't have a gold-standard to help you know how worried you should be, so you'd be acting on uncertain information.

Now let's consider that we want to find patterns between aspects of our waking life and aspects of our sleep. This usually means keeping a diary to track various things about our sleep experience, like how long it takes to fall asleep, how much total sleep has occurred, the number of awakenings we experience during the night, and so on. Traditionally this would be done by self-report, but with the availability of sleep-monitoring devices, we might use such trackers instead of the old-fashioned diary approach. We might want to do both, in case differences show up between how sleep feels and what the measurements say.[d] Tracking our waking life can also be done

---

c See chapter 8 for more on the disconnect between sleep apnea symptoms and sleep apnea measurements.

d See chapter 17 for more on sleep perception.

with old-fashioned diary entries, though more and more options are coming along that automatically track certain things like activity levels. Some of the most common factors or experiences during the day that might affect our sleep include caffeine, alcohol, exercise, napping, and stress. Diary tracking, with or without an objective monitor, can help answer common questions like "How does the amount or timing of caffeine intake affect my sleep?" This direction of "causes" has a flip side as well, since the quantity or quality of sleep could affect next-day behaviors. Caffeine is a good example: after a poor night's sleep, we might use more caffeine the next day to counteract our subsequent sleepiness. In other words, sleep quality or quantity can be seen as both "cause" and "effect" relative to our daytime experiences. If self-tracking and pattern discovery sound interesting to you, then more details await in chapter 19.

We can't bring people into the sleep lab simply to check the accuracy of their latest tracker. The trend lately toward home sleep-apnea kits is making the laboratory polysomnogram harder to get approved for medical testing. But given the known factors that can influence sensors—and the fact that consumer trackers have not been extensively studied across the range of medical problems and medications, or even with caffeine, alcohol, or nicotine—this all means that uncertainty will prevail. A person might be willing to accept uncertainty and try to use sleep trackers to improve her sleep. My main concern is that many people might be using trackers without appreciating this uncertainty, and that disconnect can create potential problems. If you look at the marketing claims of many consumer devices, it's easy to think that validation has occurred[38] despite the many critiques of the devices by sleep researchers.[39-42] That disconnect can be solved with better algorithms in the future, but in the meantime, we must at least be aware of the potential risks of interpreting consumer sleep tracking devices from a health perspective.

CHAPTER 5

My sleep is fine—why do you ask?

I have no symptoms, and I don't want to go looking for trouble

This is a very understandable sentiment, and certain health-care decisions fall into this category. For example, if a test is risky or costly, or if the disease we're talking about is not treatable, then some people might reasonably conclude that they should leave well enough alone. Other people might still seek testing, because knowledge of a disease status might be important to certain life choices or might allow them to participate in research that could help make advances for better treatment options in the future. Like all health-care decisions, we must consider a balance of potential risks and potential benefits, and we all weigh them in our own way. Let's look at two common sleep problems: sleep apnea and periodic limb movements of sleep. Each of these may or may not cause symptoms.

For sleep apnea, we can think about the question of how worried we should be in two parts. First, we can make a guess about the risk of having this problem. How do we do that? We look to the evidence from different clinical studies for the major risk factors involved. Some of those risk factors are symptoms, like snoring, gasping, or sleepiness, but these may not be the strongest clues that sleep apnea is present. It turns out that certain health problems are even more strongly associated with sleep apnea than those symptoms. Because of this finding, most screening questionnaires include people's health information in addition to their subjective symptoms. The second part of the question is: If you have sleep apnea, then how severe is the case? It turns out that severity is important for shaping how worried we should be as well as what treatment options will make most sense for us.

Even with today's growing awareness of sleep apnea as a common disorder, some people are not aware of all the treatment options beyond CPAP masks (short for "continuous positive airway pressure"). And if such people decline testing for sleep apnea by saying, "I could never wear the mask, so what's the point?" then we would want to at least bring up the various other treatment options so that they could make the decision based on more complete information. They might also refuse the other options, of course![a]

For PLMS (short for "periodic limb movements of sleep"), the situation is far less clear. If you're the type to wait for the results of large clinical trials before seeking treatment, then you wouldn't be very motivated to care about leg twitches while you sleep unless they were causing some symptoms. But if you're the type to be concerned about the research studies that have reported that PLMS is associated with health risks like heart attack and stroke,[43,44] then you might want to at least know what your numbers look like.[b] You're thinking about PLMS might be swayed if placed into the context of other health problems. Let's say you're a smoker, and you've been thinking about quitting but haven't been motivated because you're otherwise "in perfect health." I'm not saying that this is a good way to think about smoking (!), but maybe if you learned that you had elevated limb movements during sleep, then you might recalibrate your reasoning and think harder about quitting, since you now have another potential cardiovascular risk factor to consider.

How can the field of sleep medicine be so noncommittal about the reported health risks of leg movements? There are two main reasons we are not generally more aggressive about treating them in the absence of sleep symptoms. One is that we're not sure whether the associated risks are merely correlations. If so, treating the leg movements would not be expected to improve health. If, on the other hand, the health risks were actually causal, not just correlation, then we might be more willing to consider therapy for PLMS even if a person had no awareness or symptoms. Unfortunately, no studies to date have proved that our current treatments to reduce PLMS would also be effective at reducing the associated health risks.

---

a See chapters 10 and 11 for more on CPAP and other treatments for sleep apnea.

b See chapter 16 for more on PLMS.

The differential diagnosis of feeling fine

One of the first lessons in medical school is to make a list of possibilities that could explain any given symptom. This is called the differential diagnosis or just "differential." It's not just a mental exercise: as the old adage goes, if you didn't think of it, then you can't diagnose it. If a patient arrives with belly pain, then you perform a combination of talking, examining, and ordering tests to zero in on the most likely reason for belly pain from your differential diagnosis list. Maybe appendicitis was already near the top of the list, but it was important to rule out other problems that could also cause belly pain (especially those that would not be cured by surgically removing a normal appendix!).

Making a differential diagnosis list for "feeling fine" seems less intuitive. The closest analogy in health care would be to think about the logic behind screening tests. Instead of us reacting to a new symptom, screening tests aim to catch problems before they cause symptoms. Screening makes the most sense when reliable tests exist for problems that are better treated when caught early. Many adults undergo regular screening for everything from high blood pressure to different kinds of cancer. Certain sleep problems fit somewhere in between, and we'll unpack some of the ways to think about this in the next sections. We'll follow the approach of the differential diagnosis in order to think through common situations where a person with a sleep disorder could still feel fine. Like the person with belly pain who benefits from knowing what is *not* causing it, people who feel fine about their sleep might feel "even more fine" if they also knew a sleep disorder was *not* hiding under the surface.

Under the radar

Changes that are gradual and occur over long periods of time can fly under the radar of our attention. Sometimes clues pop up, like clothes no longer buttoning properly after gradual weight gain. This can happen for sleep as well, and sometimes in a quite frightening and dangerous manner, like when a person who's been gradually developing sleep apnea over many years ends up dozing off not just in the recliner while watching TV but also while behind the wheel of a car. When these kinds of accidents happen, we are startled into action, and we'll likely become aggressive about pursuing treatment. But could we have recognized the problem before catastrophe struck? If someone has—and recognizes—major problems with sleepiness, then perhaps he would be more likely to look into potential sleep disorders. But it is not so obvious for those with mild sleepiness, or symptoms that are so gradual that they fly under the radar.

Compensatory countermeasures

This category, of using techniques to compensate for sleepiness, is related to the under-the-radar category. We may find ourselves gradually, over many years, changing certain behaviors that are compensating for a gradual worsening of sleep quality. Maybe we have found that we need more sleep over time. Because there are so many potential reasons for this, we may or may not think of a primary underlying sleep disorder if we're also thinking of things like stress, family demands, or simply "getting older." We may have found that our caffeine intake has been creeping up over time, eventually becoming every day and maybe multiple servings per day. Putting aside the potential risks and benefits of coffee for the moment, the gradual change over time could be compensating or "masking" a gradually developing primary sleep problem. We can imagine a similar story for increasing naps over time. Caffeine, naps, and catch-up sleep are the main countermeasures for sleep loss that happens more quickly, like pulling an all-nighter or working a night shift without having slept the prior day. When we use such countermeasures in those settings, the reason is immediately obvious. But when countermeasure behaviors are changing very slowly over time, we may not immediately think of a sleep problem causing this to happen, especially if other competing explanations are involved.

Misattributions

This category is about the potential for unintended consequences of well-intended decisions. Sleep difficulties come in many forms, and, likewise, feeling tired during the day can have many causes. Sometimes we attribute either the sleep disturbance or the tiredness to another cause, which can distract us from looking into measuring sleep directly, especially if treating that other issue actually helps with our sleep disturbance. Let's look at a few examples.

Say you begin to notice that you have to use the bathroom during the night more and more, which is bothersome because of the sleep interruption. You may decide to look into medication treatments for this problem (called nocturia), or you may reduce your fluid intake before bedtime, or you might just chalk it up to getting older. You might find that medication or reducing fluids improves the situation, and since you're getting up less, you might not consider whether measuring sleep directly could be helpful. Sleep apnea and nocturia are both common, so they could happen together by pure chance. But one theory is that anything that disrupts sleep (like sleep apnea) can increase nocturia by keeping sleep light enough that bladder sensations reach conscious awareness. Certain sleep problems like sleep apnea can be associated with a wide range of non-sleep symptoms, such as morning headaches, acid reflux, erectile dysfunction, and high blood pressure. Even depressed mood and attention problems can be caused or worsened by untreated sleep apnea. Sometimes people are treated successfully for these other issues, but over time the issue comes back, and maybe they'll investigate sleep problems at that later time. If sleep apnea is found at that point, then we'll wonder how far back it was present and if treating the hidden breathing problem could have helped the situation.

Insomnia may be the most concerning example of potential misattribution. We may not think of sleep apnea and insomnia as going together, but the overlap is quite common.[45-48] So common, in fact, that some studies have found markedly increased rates of sleep apnea in patients with "just" insomnia, meaning that the patients showed no clues about the sleep apnea such as obesity or snoring or gasping. For those with chronic insomnia who end up taking medication for sleep, one concern is that the medication is masking (or even worsening) a hidden case of sleep apnea.

Resilience

Some people seem to be able to roll with whatever life throws at them. In neurology, we often talk about the concept of "brain reserve" to describe the common observation that even for major problems like stroke, some people have fewer symptoms than others, or a faster recovery than others, despite having similar-looking brain-scan results. The effect of sleep loss on waking function and symptoms is well-known to vary substantially from person to person.[49] Likewise, the symptoms of sleep apnea can be strikingly variable, and many don't feel sleepy at all (as we'll discuss more in chapter 8). They are not simply in denial or unaware because, even when tested for sleepiness objectively in a sleep lab, they score in the normal range. We don't yet understand why two people with the same severity of sleep apnea might have anything from zero to severe sleepiness. This theme—that people have different vulnerability versus resilience to altered physiology—permeates all aspects of health, and sleep is no exception.

CHAPTER 6

I need some tips to help me sleep

What is sleep hygiene?

The usual tips to help people sleep typically come in the form of a series of "do" and "don't" bullet points collectively known by the somewhat unfortunate term "sleep hygiene." The American Academy of Sleep Medicine recommends these topics in its "Clinical Guideline for the Evaluation and Management of Chronic Insomnia in Adults."[50] Here are a few common examples of sleep-hygiene tips:

Do:

> keep the bedroom quiet and dark and cool
> get up at the same time every day
> go to bed only when sleepy
> have a bedtime relaxation plan or ritual
> get out of bed and do something relaxing if you've been awake for over twenty minutes
> exercise, but not too close to bedtime

Don't:

> go to bed hungry, but also don't eat too close to bedtime
> consume alcohol too close to bedtime (three to four hours)
> have nicotine too close to bedtime (one to two hours)
> consume caffeine after lunch
> view bright lights or electronics right before bed nap after 3:00 p.m. (and if you do nap, keep it to less than thirty to sixty minutes)

Does sleep hygiene really work?

These seem like common-sense tips that would be helpful. But in the spirit of healthy debate, let's jump right into some perspective the academy has provided about sleep hygiene: "Although all patients with chronic insomnia should adhere to rules of good sleep hygiene, there is insufficient evidence to indicate that sleep hygiene alone is effective in the treatment of chronic insomnia. It should be used in combination with other therapies." The academy's recommendations for sleep hygiene are what we call "consensus," meaning that the expert panel writing the guidelines agrees with sleep hygiene in general, but research evidence supporting the recommendations is lacking.

It may seem counterintuitive that the collective opinions of leaders within a field can be considered a weak form of evidence. It may also seem like sleep-hygiene tips are so common sense and obvious that we don't need research studies to prove that they are effective. But in the era of evidence-based medicine, even straightforward topics like this are subject to rigorous testing, and in the case of sleep hygiene, the research turns out to be thin. But the weak-evidence basis should not be interpreted as evidence that these tips don't matter for sleep. Instead, it seems reasonable to think about sleep hygiene as a first level of options. Some may find the tips helpful, while others won't enjoy much benefit from them. Depending on the situation, we may want to continue our efforts at tidying up these hygiene topics even if by themselves they aren't launching a person into successful slumber, if only to remove barriers so that a next level of treatment is more likely to succeed. Treatments like cognitive behavioral therapy (CBT) for insomnia incorporate sleep hygiene directly as part of a more comprehensive approach to improving sleep.[a] For someone who did not improve with sleep hygiene alone and ends up taking a sleeping pill for insomnia, we would still want to stack the deck in favor of sleep by making good sleep-hygiene choices so that the medication doesn't have to fight an uphill battle.

What does it mean to put these tips into context?

The role of context is in helping everyone figure out where to put their energy and how to prioritize different aspects of sleep hygiene. After reviewing the list of possible tips, picking the top choices to focus on could depend on what's feasible given individual work or family constraints, or what is most likely to be a root cause based on

---

a See chapter 14 for more on CBT for insomnia.

past experience. Let's unpack a few of them to shed light on how even a harmless or easy-sounding tip might not make sense for everyone to implement.

Caffeine: This age-old chemical is a double-edged sword of competing issues to consider. First and foremost we have the energy boost that some people derive from coffee. We must balance this benefit against the potential risk of sleep disturbance or other adverse effects of the caffeine (headache, acid reflux, and so forth). While some may view this as a simple example of "all things in moderation," we can make it more personalized by rephrasing the question: How much in the way of side effects or sleep disturbance would you be willing to tolerate for the benefits you identify from caffeine? The differences in caffeine response from person to person can be dramatic, whether we're looking at real-world experience or even carefully controlled research studies,[51] some of which we now know are due to genetic differences.[52] These topics exist in the context of cultural and taste preferences, which to some extent can be flexible if we are willing to consider decaffeinated options.

Naps: Here we also have a double-edged sword of risks and benefits, and perhaps even more individual variability than occurs with caffeine. Ask a roomful of adults how many of them can nap, and of those, how many feel refreshed as if from a power nap, and you'll not only see the variety of personal experience with naps, but you'll also see a few sideways glances from those who are thinking, "Who has time to nap?" For those who can nap, the timing within the day, the duration of the nap—even details like body position (chair versus couch versus bed), light exposure, and temperature—these and other factors may influence how you feel upon awakening. How much you have slept recently also plays an important role: if you've been running a sleep debt over the past night or two, then it might be easier to nap, but you might notice yourself craving more than just a power nap to feel caught up. For those who cannot seem to nap at all, just lying down to physically rest may be refreshing, even if sleep doesn't enter the equation. We need to balance the potential benefits of napping to increase energy against the potential downside of the nap interfering with nighttime sleep. The inner clock that keeps track of recent sleep (the homeostat[b]) can become confused if a nap is too long or is taken too late in the day, making the brain less willing to welcome slumber when bedtime comes around.

Exercise: For the average person, exercise is energizing and best done earlier in the day. It seems to make good sense to keep it early if exercise leaves you feeling activated

---

b See chapter 15 for more on the two inner clocks, circadian and homeostatic, that control sleep-wake rhythms.

or energetic, and thus you would find it harder to wind down and fall asleep if you exercised later, especially if light exposure during exercise exacerbates this effect. But is this tip equally important for everyone? The National Sleep Foundation suggests that individuals may differ in their response to exercise, and that people should figure out the timing that works best for them.[53] Maybe some people feel tired after working out, and some find that exercise helps to blow off steam or reduce anxious thoughts that could interfere with sleep. In those cases, exercising later in the day or even at night might seem more natural. What if a person only has time to exercise in the evening, and it doesn't seem to bother her ability to sleep—in such a situation, should she adhere strictly to the tip of no exercise at night if the alternative were not to exercise at all? Even more interesting to consider is the person who chooses evening exercise but experiences mild insomnia symptoms; might a reasonable person still choose the overall benefit of regular exercise as a worthwhile trade-off? This is the idea of context, illustrated by an example of competing interests. In this case, one recommendation of "don't exercise at night to avoid hurting sleep" meets another recommendation of "regular exercise is good for health."

Getting out of bed after twenty minutes of being awake: I don't always recommend this hygiene tip to patients with chronic insomnia. Two competing ideas need to be balanced here. Staying in bed and getting more and more frustrated about being awake can actually make it even harder to fall back asleep. Over time, this experience can actually perpetuate the insomnia pattern, and thus we have the root of the recommendation to get out of bed. However, getting out of bed brings its own risk by increasing the chance of being exposed to wake-promoting factors and could perpetuate insomnia over time. Examples of things that could confuse the sleep system once you are out of bed include exposure to light, food, and social media, and even standing upright can be a wake-promoting factor. Following the twenty-minute tip can lead to clock-watching, which itself can worsen insomnia symptoms. Another twist relates to sleep perception: we know from many studies that we may be getting sleep even when we feel awake (that is, until we get out of bed).[c] For those who are able to remain calm, the alternative to the twenty-minute tip is to remain in bed with the relaxing combination of being horizontal, lying in the dark, and breathing comfortably. Each person can think about which option seems more sensible or tolerable from their experience. Their answer might even be different from night to night—that's OK, too.

---

c See chapter 17 for more on the perception of sleep.

Although some might be reassured of having a plan firmly in place every night, for others, knowing that options exist may take the edge off.

Going to bed only when sleepy: This seems reasonable, but I usually offer a few conditions to help give this tip more bang for its buck. The benefit of this tip is that it provides some flexibility about bedtime, because forcing yourself into bed when you're not tired is a setup for frustration and could prolong the time it takes to fall asleep. On the other hand, for those who are high-energy people who don't have a reasonable plan for wind-down time in preparation for bed, or even a target bedtime in mind, then waiting until they feel tired could mean hours of awake time later than intended, especially if they're engaged in some interesting activity at night. Striking a balance is important—and the act of winding down, dimming the lights, and even getting horizontal instead of vertical can be calming and help usher in sleep.

Finally, although it is standard practice to use sleep diaries to track patterns, with the goal of improving sleep habits and getting better sleep, even this core clinical technique might backfire for some. If pulling out the diary to record each awakening is frustrating, or if it means you're looking at the clock to record a time, or if you're turning the light on to do any of this, then the act of keeping the diary could be inadvertently contributing to insomnia. Consider people with obsessive compulsive disorder—the task of keeping a diary might increase their anxiety levels and make their insomnia worse.

Beyond trial and error

Figuring out which of these tips will or won't work seems simple enough: just a little trial and error sprinkled in with some thoughtful reflection on prior personal experiences. When following a sleep tip has a very strong effect (good or bad), it is easy to draw meaningful personal conclusions. But for many people, the effects of any one sleep tip will likely be small, and in the real world, where a lot can happen in a given day that could affect sleep, we might need to try a tip for more than just one night to be sure we understand the effects. External factors, individual differences in sleep and wake habits, and how many nights are necessary to maintain a behavior all remain important challenges for self-discovery.[d] Trial and error might mean trying different tips on different days. Maybe some people can only meditate when they're in the right frame of mind, which might differ from night to night. Forcing such a person

---

d See chapter 19 for more on self-discovery.

into a strict routine could backfire. Rather, it seems better to think of hygiene tips as a palette of options from which to choose, based on a personal sense of what is most natural or most likely to work. How you feel about your sleep now can shape the approach to sleep hygiene. For someone who's healthy and feels good about his sleep but is trying to be mindful, trying the hygiene tips alone or in combination might help him discover which ones, if any, seem to make a tangible impact on his well-being. For the chronic insomnia patient, it might make more sense to think of hygiene tips as part of a bigger picture. Insomnia can be quite challenging to wrangle, as a huge number of factors could potentially be involved.[e] Rather than thinking of the whole list of sleep-hygiene tips as mandatory therapy, thinking of the list as several small battlefronts makes them easier to place into context and decide where to put one's energy. If we just hand people sleep tips in isolation and don't help them work through decisions in their own context, then we are arguably focusing too much on the trees and missing an opportunity to see the forest and engage the big picture for making decisions and behavior changes that will stick.

---

e See chapters 12 and 13 for more on insomnia.

CHAPTER 7

I feel tired even when I do get enough sleep

What's the difference between sleepiness and fatigue?

Sleepiness and fatigue sound like they could mean the same thing, or least something very similar to each other. If feeling tired is yet a third kind of experience, is it closer to feeling sleepy or closer to feeling fatigued? Does non-refreshing sleep mean something different yet again? Will teasing these questions apart case by case lead us to different diagnostic testing or treatment options? That there are no clear answers may seem a little unsatisfying, in part because people may use the terms interchangeably when describing their personal experiences, and in part because we don't have good objective tests to distinguish them either. When I ask patients in my clinic about these things, I try to provide examples to set sleepiness and fatigue as different ends of a spectrum. If sleepiness means the tendency or actual experience of falling asleep at an unwanted time, and fatigue means having low energy or feeling tired, but you wouldn't fall asleep even if you lay down, then which is closer to your experience? Thinking through the symptoms can help provide context for tracking improvements as we undertake treatment options. Overnight polysomnography testing in the sleep laboratory[a] can shed light on the potential causes of daytime symptoms (whether a person describes sleepiness or fatigue), such as sleep apnea or periodic limb movements of sleep, which we'll talk about in the next section. Daytime testing, with repeated nap opportunities, is generally considered a test of sleepiness because it measures how fast a person is able to fall asleep if given the opportunity to do so. In clinical sleep medicine practice, no reliable diagnostic tests have yet been proven to quantify fatigue objectively.

---

a See chapter 18 for more on sleep diagnostics.

We can also consider the question of whether feeling sleepy or fatigued during the day necessarily has anything to do with sleep. These feelings are what we call non-specific, meaning they could be caused by any number of health problems, or from medication side effects, or even a psychiatric disorder like depression. Usually by the time a person with these symptoms reaches a specialty sleep clinic, the usual suspects of nonsleep-related causes have been investigated and ruled out. Common testing methods include blood counts for anemia, liver and kidney function tests, blood sugar levels, and thyroid hormone levels. The fact that fatigue, sleepiness, and tiredness are nonspecific means that the possible causes include disorders of sleep as well as general medical problems and psychiatric disorders. Keeping an open mind to these different categories, and understanding the context of each person's story case by case, can help us to prioritize decisions about testing and help us focus on points of improvement if we pursue treatments.

Which sleep disorders most commonly cause sleepiness?

This might seem like a strange question—don't all sleep disorders cause sleepiness? Theoretically, the answer is yes: just about anything that interferes with sleep can potentially cause sleepiness during the day. Surprisingly, however, the links between sleepiness and sleep disorders are actually quite variable from person to person. Sleep apnea is a prime example. This is a disorder of breathing that causes interruptions of airflow repeatedly while a person sleeps, often accompanied by drops in oxygen levels and other changes in physiology that signify stress and increased adrenaline-system activity. Despite these dramatic changes and disruptions to the normal calmness of sleep cycling, so many adults with sleep apnea have no sleepiness that we'll spend a whole chapter exploring this disconnect between symptoms and disease severity.[b] Insomnia is another common sleep problem, and you'd think that struggling to fall asleep or stay asleep at night would directly cause increased sleepiness during the day. In fact, for the typical patient with chronic insomnia, the opposite happens: patients actually experience less than average sleepiness during the day when measured with objective testing.[c] This unexpected observation led to the proposal of chronic insomnia as a disorder of hyperarousal[54] that affects people twenty-four hours a day. Chronic insomnia not only interferes with nighttime sleep but also negatively affects daytime

---

b See chapter 8 for more on sleep apnea and sleepiness.

c See chapter 18 for more on sleep diagnostics.

function while reducing the chance for catch-up sleep. Some patients refer to this experience as feeling "wired but tired."

Sleepiness due to insufficient sleep quantity or quality

It is probably the case that the most common cause of sleepiness in adults is simply insufficient sleep due to nonmedical reasons, meaning that either work or personal obligations (or both) are cutting into the time people usually set aside for sleep. A number of medical and psychiatric disorders can affect the quantity of sleep as well. Common examples include chronic pain, bladder problems, acid reflux, or heart problems, any of which can interfere with the amount of sleep we obtain and, as we'll see in the next section, could also interfere with the quality of the sleep we get. Medications may have side effects that reduce sleep quantity, though it is more common for medications to cause drowsiness as a direct side effect or indirectly by interfering with sleep quality. The experience of reduced sleep quantity, regardless of the cause, may seem to resemble insomnia, in the sense that people have difficulty either falling asleep or staying asleep. But chronic insomnia is not typically associated with daytime sleepiness, even when objectively measured in nap studies, despite patients sometimes reporting severe reductions in total amount of sleep.

The two most common sleep disorders that impair sleep quality involve abnormal breathing or abnormal muscle twitches. The rhythmic leg twitches known as periodic limb movements of sleep (PLMS) are related to restless legs syndrome, both of which we'll discuss further in chapter 16. Sleep apnea, which is the most common breathing disorder during sleep, is associated with repeated interruptions in breathing. The main subtype is obstructive sleep apnea, in which the problem is caused by intermittent collapse of the soft tissue at the back of the throat, which then leads to temporary blockages of airflow. A less common form of sleep apnea, known as central sleep apnea, is associated with interruptions in breathing despite having an open airway due to abnormalities in the neural reflexes that control breathing during sleep. Although we might expect such frightening-sounding interruptions of sleep to cause daytime sleepiness, it turns out that only about half of patients with sleep apnea, including those with severe cases, experience daytime sleepiness as a result. Despite this disconnect between symptoms and disease severity, it is important to consider sleep apnea as a potential root cause of sleepiness in the hope of reversing the symptoms by diagnosing and treating the sleep apnea.

Sleepiness despite normal nighttime sleep measurements

Performing overnight polysomnography testing in the sleep lab is the gold-standard method for diagnosing sleep apnea, periodic limb movements, and other less common causes of impaired sleep quality. But even this advanced testing cannot detect certain sleep disorders, known as primary or "central" causes of sleepiness. The two most common forms are narcolepsy and idiopathic hypersomnia (the latter of which means sleepiness of unknown cause). Narcolepsy as a cause of sleepiness is usually suspected based on the presence of three other symptoms that have their roots in the physiology of dreaming intruding into wakefulness. Sleep paralysis is the experience of the inability to move (usually as one is just waking up from sleep), which can last a minute or two and may be very frightening. Sleep-onset hallucinations refer to dream-like experiences, often visual in nature, which people have just before sleep begins while they are still awake. Cataplexy is a sudden loss of muscle strength that is triggered by laughter (and sometimes other emotions). This can affect parts of the body such as the face or one arm, or it can involve the entire body, resulting in a person collapsing to the ground (they appear asleep because they cannot move, but they are in fact awake). People with narcolepsy typically have normal measurements of sleep during overnight polysomnogram testing but show abnormalities during a battery of daytime nap blocks called a multiple sleep latency test (or MSLT).[d] During a series of four or five opportunities to nap spread throughout the day, people with narcolepsy fall asleep faster than normal, and they are more likely to enter dream (REM) sleep during the naps. These physiological measurements reflect the core features of narcolepsy: sleepiness, as indicated by the rapid onset of sleep during the nap opportunities, and, once asleep, entering REM sleep abnormally fast.

Idiopathic hypersomnia shares the excessive sleepiness symptoms present in people with narcolepsy, but it differs from narcolepsy in that it does not cause the intrusion of dreamlike experiences. When testing people for idiopathic hypersomnia, the MSLT shows abnormally fast onset of sleep during the nap opportunities but no excess REM sleep during the naps. As in the case of narcolepsy, the results of the overnight polysomnogram testing in idiopathic hypersomnia cases are typically normal.

Unlike the treatment strategies for sleep apnea and periodic limb movements, which focus on reversing the root cause, the treatments for narcolepsy and idiopathic hypersomnia are geared toward symptom relief. This often involves the prescription

---

d See chapter 18 for more on sleep diagnostic testing, including the MSLT.

of stimulant medications to counteract the sleepiness. Taking naps, ingesting caffeine, and keeping a regular sleep schedule can also be helpful for some people. For the REM intrusion symptoms that occur with narcolepsy, medications such as antidepressants that suppress REM sleep can be helpful. Although research studies have shown that some patients with narcolepsy and cataplexy are deficient in a neurochemical called orexin as the root cause, we do not yet have treatments to correct this deficiency. The neurochemical basis of idiopathic hypersomnia remains unclear, but research in the last 5 years or so has raised the possibility that in some patients, the brain produces a chemical similar to a class of sedative medications called benzodiazepines (an example is diazepam, one brand of which is Valium).[55]

CHAPTER 8

How can I have sleep apnea if I feel fine?

Don't just listen to your body; make it a two-way conversation

t might seem natural to think that if you feel fine when you wake up, you have no complaints about sleep, and you have good energy during the day, what more could you ask for than to reach this little taste of nocturnal nirvana? Why would we even look for problems in such a person? This is the "if it ain't broke, don't fix it" mentality. This mentality makes sense sometimes. What we need to understand is how all of us can be confident that our sleep "ain't broke" based solely on experience.

Come on, I don't even snore!

I never thought during the early years of my neurology training that I'd find my future self involved in marriage counseling. But the bedroom is an interesting ecosystem, and interesting perspectives are often revealed in my sleep clinic for people who sleep with a bed partner. Sometimes a worried spouse describes her nights of watching anxiously for signs of stopped breathing. Sometimes the bed partner reports such loud snoring that even the ear plugs that were a successful parry in prior years are no longer a match for the noise. When it comes to sleep apnea, the two major medical concerns are daytime symptoms and long-term health risks. But a third category of concern exists for thinking about how worried we should be about sleep apnea: bed-partner happiness. It can be incredibly frustrating for concerned family members—who are also suffering sleep disturbance from the noise of snoring and the anxious surveillance for breathing problems—to find their concern meets with denial of snoring (or even snarky replies like "You're the one who snores!"). More than once in my sleep clinic, a spouse has been waiting, almost as if in ambush, for the denial of snoring, at which point the spouse produces exhibit A with fanfare—a recording of the alleged crime! Likewise, more than once, the alleged snorer has provocatively asked me whether the swift elbow in the ribs multiple times per night from the bed partner might itself be hurting sleep quality more than the snoring.

Let's unpack the scene here for a moment. The spouse is rightfully frustrated: How can people be so sure they aren't snoring? If you were asleep, how would you know one way or the other? It's an interesting question.[a] Maybe it's just an instinct to deny it, either because it's embarrassing or because we just don't want to be bothered. Sometimes people think they aren't asleep in the first place, like when my grandpa would sit on the recliner in front of the TV, doze off, start snoring, and then pop awake when we changed the channel, upset about the channel changing and the "you were snoring" explanation. Even when the spouse or family says, "Look, we're the ones who hear you snoring like a chainsaw every night, while you sleep through your own roaring," the patient may still resist. And the family may be thinking: Let's get real here, which is more likely, that you're actually snoring, or that we're inventing stories to trick you into getting a sleep test and wearing a sleep mask? From this perspective, we might even look at a person who has symptoms—say, gasping during sleep—as "lucky," in the sense that we have one less barrier to overcome on the road to diagnosis and treatment.

How refreshed we feel during the day is also worth a closer look. This feeling is shaped by many factors and can be hard to describe, let alone formally measure in a clinic or in a research study. Thinking about the range of possibilities can provide important context. Could a lack of sleepiness be from true resilience to sleep loss, or is sleepiness present but being masked by countermeasures like naps or caffeine? How concerned we might be can relate to how the sleepiness affects daily life: a long work meeting and a long drive in the car might be equally boring, but dozing off has very different consequences in these two situations. An entire chapter (chapter 5) is devoted to the question of how we can think about sleep when it feels fine.

Sleep apnea is a chameleon

Ask people about sleep apnea, and the response could be anywhere from "What's that?" to "That's a deadly disease that causes heart attacks and car accidents and

---

a See chapter 17 for more on disconnects between how sleep feels and what sleep measurements reveal.

dementia." That range of perspectives is about as broad as the disease itself, which can range from so mild that we're not sure it warrants treatment to so severe that we might even think about surgical therapies. Just as disease severity is variable on objective testing, so can the subjective experience of symptoms range from barely noticeable to crippling sleepiness that affects daily life. It might seem surprising that experiencing repeated episodes of not breathing throughout the night doesn't *always* cause symptoms and problems. Some may gasp so strongly or snore so loudly that they wake themselves up during the night. Even people who wake with these symptoms might only feel them occasionally, whereas the interruptions in breathing that occur in sleep apnea are happening many more times per hour during sleep. Some people with sleep apnea don't have the smoking-gun symptoms of snoring and gasping and daytime sleepiness but instead might have more indirect symptoms, like headache, or mood changes, or reduced sexual function. Because these daytime symptoms have many potential causes, they might not immediately make anyone think of sleep apnea. Once we recognize that sleep apnea can cause different symptoms in different people, we can better understand how to think about sleep apnea in context.

The most surprising end of this wide spectrum of symptoms of sleep apnea is that some people have no symptoms at all. Still more surprising is just how common this disconnect turns out to be: it's not just a small portion of super-resilient people who manage to tolerate breathing interruptions without sleepiness. Two research studies make this point nicely by reporting unexpectedly high proportions of sleep apnea discovered in carefully selected groups of people with no sleep complaints. One study from 2008 was of healthy non-obese adults[56] and another from 2017 was of older adults in good general health and with normal cognitive testing.[57] If we look just at people who have been diagnosed with a severe case of sleep apnea, only about half of them report sleepiness, whether by being asked survey questions or by being testing objectively in the sleep laboratory with a nap-testing protocol.[b] But the thought that poor sleep from sleep apnea must cause non-refreshing sleep and sleepiness is so strong that in the early days of sleep medicine (in the 1980s and 1990s), a patient had to have symptoms such as sleepiness before the doctor would make the diagnosis of sleep apnea. This meant that, no matter how many times people stop breathing during sleep, or how low their oxygen dropped, they didn't have the disease of sleep apnea if they were not sleepy. In current clinical practice, we no longer follow this

---

b See chapter 18 for more on diagnostic testing.

rather extreme stance, and nor do we follow the opposite extreme: that everyone with sleep apnea, no matter how mild the case, requires treatment.

When we measure sleep apnea, the condition can seem so disruptive and dramatic that it is hard to believe anyone could sleep through it, not to mention waking up refreshed as if nothing were wrong. Worse still, we can't yet predict, even with all our diagnostic measurements, whether any given person will feel sleepy or non-refreshed. Perhaps this is not so surprising if we take a step back and remember that we can't even predict whether people are going to feel like they were asleep or awake during the night of polysomnogram testing.[c] It could be that we are not measuring sleep apnea severity as well as we could. Maybe some detail about the breathing, or the oxygen level, or the brain waves, holds the clues, if only we could measure these details more precisely. Or maybe we all have our own sensitivities to the effects of sleep apnea, like how different people have different pain thresholds.

Does everyone with sleep apnea need treatment?

The decision to undergo treatment for sleep apnea requires that we think about two aspects of the disease: (1) the severity based on objective diagnostic testing[d] and (2) the symptoms and health status of the individual. This fits nicely into the repeated need to consider context. The American Academy of Sleep Medicine directly addresses the need for this combined thinking in its practice guidelines.[58] If the case of sleep apnea is mild, meaning that the apnea-hypopnea index (AHI) is between five and fifteen breathing interruptions per hour of sleep, then treatment should be considered if sleep-related symptoms are present or if other medical disorders that could be affected by untreated sleep apnea, like high blood pressure, are present. The guidelines recognize that symptoms could mean more than sleepiness, and they even mention having insomnia as reason enough to pursue treatment for mild sleep apnea.[e] For sleep apnea cases with AHI values in the moderate range (fifteen to thirty events per hour of sleep) or severe range (more than thirty events per hour of sleep), treatment is recommended even if people have no symptoms, because the health risks are more likely at these severity levels.

---

c See chapter 17 for more on the perception of sleep.

d See chapters 9 and 18 for more on at-home and in-lab diagnostic testing.

e See chapter 13 for more on the overlap between insomnia and sleep apnea.

This approach is a way to balance objective and subjective data in order to determine how worried we should be. The evolution of thinking about sleep apnea is in part because of research on the health risks of untreated sleep apnea, including heart disease, high blood pressure, and motor vehicle accidents. It turns out that the risks are linked to sleep apnea severity, and the most accepted measure of severity is the AHI value obtained from diagnostic testing. The health risks are stronger for moderate cases compared to mild cases, and strongest of all for severe cases of sleep apnea.

Just when you thought that approach seems reasonable, the latest studies (as of early 2018) have put a twist on current thinking about sleep apnea. The twist seems like a throwback to the traditional thinking that required symptoms of sleepiness to make the diagnosis of sleep apnea. One influential study in 2016 tested the effects of CPAP treatment in adults with sleep apnea who were at increased risk for heart disease but who were not particularly sleepy. The researchers found no benefit of CPAP treatment for improving heart health.[1] Needless to say, this created a stir, as many doctors and patients were using improvements in health—especially heart health—as a major motivation to treat sleep apnea with CPAP. The question of whether the absence of sleepiness signifies in some patients a kind of resistance to the cardiovascular risk of sleep apnea is still under debate. After all, this was a major study that was published in a top medical journal, and maybe those who lack sleepiness really are resistant to other health risks of sleep apnea as well. On the other hand, it seems hard to imagine that a questionnaire about the experience of sleepiness could capture something special about heart attack risk but would not correlate well with any of the many measurements we make in the sleep lab,[59,60] including the severity of sleep apnea. It also seems strange that in the same trial that did not show a heart benefit, the subjective symptoms of sleepiness and quality of life were significantly improved by CPAP treatment. Those subjective benefits occurred even though the people who participated in the study did not use their CPAP very much (under four hours per night on average). This is a reminder that adherence to CPAP is a tough challenge for many people, and in this research study, the CPAP usage might not have been enough to provide heart protection. The improvement in subjective symptoms and quality of life, despite the lack of heart benefits, is another example of the disconnects that can occur between symptoms and measurements, and is not easy to reconcile with the idea that sleepiness is biologically tied to heart risk in sleep apnea patients.

One thing is for sure: with all the uncertainty in the research about sleep apnea, it's never been more important to maintain our focus on context when making health decisions. As we mentioned earlier in the chapter, when diagnostic testing shows the sleep apnea to be mild, then the health risks are less clear, so we might need more motivation to pursue treatment, like symptoms or other health problems that might benefit from treating the sleep apnea. For moderate or severe cases of sleep apnea, the risks are stronger, which can be a stronger motivation to pursue treatment, even when symptoms are not present. The recent data we just reviewed about lack of heart protection from CPAP in those who aren't particularly sleepy should make us ask: Are we willing to take the chance of no treatment for even severe sleep apnea, just because we have no symptoms? I hope that we'll understand in the future, once we've done more research, why some patients with sleep apnea have more symptoms yet some feel fine, and how those differences relate to other health risks of this disease. Until then, simply remembering that the symptoms are not predicted by the disease severity provides important context, so we don't conclude all is well simply because of the lack of symptoms.[f]

Where does screening fit into the picture?

People come to sleep-apnea evaluation through many different paths and, as discussed earlier in this chapter, sometimes they do so against their own will. Most cases are diagnosed because either the patient noticed a problem, the patient's family members suspected a problem, or the physician found sufficient clues to recommend testing. How a person ends up in the sleep clinic provides context for decision-making based on how worried or motivated they may be. Someone who feels fine may not be as motivated to pursue testing and treatment for sleep apnea as someone who can't stay awake even during leisure activities. The person who has several health problems (such as diabetes or heart disease) that are linked to sleep apnea might be more motivated than someone who's otherwise healthy.

But what if neither symptoms nor health problems are present? The idea of screening for any disease is precisely that the disease might be developing before symptoms or health problems arise. Screening for sleep apnea would be very simple if each person with sleep apnea always snored, woke up gasping for air, and felt sleepy during the day. But as we've seen in this chapter, symptoms and even witnessed interruptions of breathing don't reliably predict sleep apnea. I would argue that no other common (yet treatable) disease remains so underdiagnosed in adults as sleep apnea. In this context, it seems that sleep apnea would be the perfect disease to develop

---

f See chapter 10 for more on CPAP treatment and chapter 11 for alternatives to CPAP.

screening programs. While sometimes this can happen, like in weight-loss surgery clinics and other specialty settings, screening has not yet enjoyed deployment in more general settings. This is in part because the screening questionnaires are not as accurate as we'd like, and even the home sleep apnea testing kits are not recommended for general screening purposes.[58] Some authorities have even argued against general sleep apnea screening because the evidence is so limited in terms of beneficial outcomes.[61]

Given these uncertainties, how are individuals to gauge how concerned they should be? We would like to be able to move beyond the old-fashioned approach of waiting for symptoms to arise before looking for sleep apnea, which we know can develop gradually over time and often without prominent symptoms. On the other hand, it is not currently feasible to perform objective diagnostic testing for sleep apnea on all adults. Again, we turn to context to provide us with some guidance for how worried we should be: How worried is my family? How worried is my doctor? How bad are my symptoms? For this third question, do I have one or more serious health problems that have been linked to untreated sleep apnea, such as heart disease or neurological disease or diabetes or high blood pressure? What would it mean to go undiagnosed for a young healthy person with mild sleep apnea but no symptoms versus an obese diabetic patient with poorly controlled high blood pressure who's already had two heart attacks? Should we be reassured if such a person felt fine, so much so that we don't consider the possibility of sleep apnea contributing to those problems?

CHAPTER 9

I had a home sleep apnea test. Now what?

n some ways, the move to home testing for sleep apnea has been a big step forward in access to diagnosis and treatment. In other ways, however, it has been an unintentional step backward by oversimplifying sleep apnea and having either limited or no ability to measure other aspects of sleep that could be important for understanding the full picture of sleep problems case by case. If sleep apnea were a single disease, and if you either had it or you didn't, and if it was the only sleep disorder worth testing for, then we'd have much less to worry about when it comes to home testing kits. In this chapter we'll see that none of those "ifs" is actually true.

Are home testing kits for everyone?

Before we talk about interpreting the results of home testing kits, let's review some pros and cons to understand their intended usage. These portable monitors have fewer sensors than a polysomnogram test conducted in a sleep laboratory. Usually patients apply the sensors from the kit themselves right before bedtime. Most of the kits include a belt around the chest to measure breathing movements, a sensor on the finger to measure oxygen levels, and thin tubing just under the nose to measure air flow. These kits have one goal: detecting sleep apnea. The interpretation of home testing data becomes less clear when we're considering other sleep disorders or if other medical problems are present that can interfere with the interpretation of home kit results.

The question about home testing kits is better framed as: What trade-offs are you willing to accept? We'll review those trade-offs in the coming sections. The "you" in that question is ideally patients, in discussion with their health-care providers, but insurance companies also weigh in on this equation, sometimes heavily. Some have argued, rightly, that the term "home sleep apnea test" (HSAT) is more appropriate than the term "home sleep test" (HST) to reflect the focus of these devices solely on the diagnosis of sleep apnea. We could argue for even more naming clarifications of these devices, but HSAT is a much easier acronym than, say, HOSATFPWOSDOCFTCI (home obstructive sleep apnea test for people without other sleep disorders or complicating factors that compromise interpretation).

Are home kits as accurate as in-lab polysomnography?

After hearing about what's involved in laboratory sleep testing, it isn't hard to imagine why many people would prefer an at-home option instead. In this way, home testing practically sells itself: it's simpler, cheaper, and faster—who wouldn't want these benefits? They seem important enough to outweigh just about any disadvantages. As in many aspects of medical care, however, the devil is in the details, and making the best decisions about sleep testing means understanding which details matter on a case-by-case basis.

It is interesting to think about how the way in which the question of accuracy is phrased can actually imply there is a simple answer. In other words, it seems like a yes-or-no kind of question. But the broken record just won't stop playing: the answer is that context matters. We'll discuss how several important trade-offs can guide our degree of confidence in home testing compared to in-lab polysomnography. We can and should be comfortable with a conclusion that what seems good or accurate on average might seem inappropriate for certain individuals. Put another way, we should think about how close a given person is to the average: to the "ideal" case of intended use of a home testing kit. The ideal situation is when (1) obstructive sleep apnea is strongly suspected, (2) no other sleep disorders are being considered, (3) no other health factors are present that could complicate interpretation, and (4) the intended treatment path is CPAP if sleep apnea is discovered. The further away people are from that ideal situation, the more attention they need to pay to the limitations of home testing. Even the supposed financial benefits, which may seem most credible, come into question when we put home testing into context.[62]

The main limitations of home testing stem from the very feature that makes them a low-cost and convenient option: they contain only a subset of the sensors usually present in a night of laboratory testing. As a result, these kits cannot detect certain sleep disorders, and the one disease the kits are intended to detect, obstructive sleep apnea, may not be detected as accurately as the in-lab polysomnogram test would (more on this in a moment).

Not being able to diagnose what we have not measured is an obvious problem. But not all sleep disorders require an objective test. Some common ones, besides sleep apnea, are worth briefly noting here (see the footnotes to get more information). We cannot diagnose periodic limb movements of sleep[a] because modern kits do not have sensors on the legs. We cannot test for parasomnias like REM behavior disorder because modern kits do not typically include the necessary brain, eye, and muscle sensors. We cannot evaluate the misperception form of insomnia[b] because most home tests do not include measurement of sleep stages. Finally, we cannot test for hypersomnia disorders[c] like narcolepsy, which also require measurement of sleep stages.

Home kits are not validated to detect other forms of breathing problems besides obstructive sleep apnea, such as central sleep apnea or a problem of low oxygen levels without sleep apnea (sometimes called hypoventilation). These limitations matter differently for different people, depending on their risk factors. For example, heavy smokers with emphysema are at risk for both sleep apnea and, independently, low oxygen levels. The same dual risk is present for individuals who are very obese. Conditions such as heart failure, certain neurological disorders, and chronic opiate medication use can each increase the risk of central sleep apnea.

For obstructive sleep apnea, it would be wonderful if this were a yes-or-no diagnostic question. But oversimplifying any disease like this comes with potential drawbacks. Research is showing that details about the sleep apnea can be important to personalize therapy, for example to predict the response to different treatment options. One of those details is also important for the decision to seek treatment or not in the first place: How severe is the case of sleep apnea? Home testing kits are known to underestimate the severity of sleep apnea. Underestimation matters differently case by case. This kind of detail could mean the difference between treatment or no treatment if the home test comes back normal but sleep apnea were actually present. Similarly, a treatment decision could hang in the balance even when the test shows sleep apnea: if the kit reports the severity is in the mild range, but has underestimated a true level

---

a See chapter 16 for more on leg movements during sleep.

b See chapter 17 for more on sleep perception.

c See chapter 7 for more on hypersomnia.

of moderate sleep apnea, then the motivation to pursue treatment might be as strong as if the true severity was known.

How likely is a home kit to underestimate sleep apnea severity? If the kit is one of the many that do not measure sleep stages, then the index of sleep apnea severity, the AHI, is reported as the number of breathing events per hour of recording, rather than per hour of sleep. Since the recording duration is always at least somewhat longer than the sleep duration, this causes underestimation of the severity index that is proportional to how much time in bed you've spent awake. If you sleep solidly, then this is less of an issue. But the more time you spend awake, the more underestimation of the sleep apnea severity. This is doubly challenging since our own estimate of sleep versus awake duration may not match well with objective measures,[d] so we can't use our own experience to help correct for this missing information. The American Academy of Sleep Medicine guidelines note that home kits should not be used to detect sleep apnea in those with prominent insomnia because of this potential for underestimation from not measuring sleep duration objectively and using recording duration instead.

The other reason sleep apnea severity might be underestimated relates to body position, which is only measured in certain home testing kits. Most breathing problems like sleep apnea are worse when sleeping on the back (supine position) compared to sleeping on the side (lateral position). For some people, the difference by position is so prominent that the breathing problem occurs only when sleeping supine. If a sleep testing kit returns with a normal result, unless we had also measured body position we would not know for sure if it was truly normal even while sleeping supine, or if it only appeared normal because no sleep had occurred in the supine position on that night.

What if the home test is negative for sleep apnea?

Now that we've seen some of the pros and cons, we can get back to practical questions and real-world decision-making. We learned in the previous section about some of the reasons a home testing kit might underestimate sleep apnea severity. When the home test is normal, this could be due to underestimation of what was really a mild or even moderate case. Even severe cases can be underestimated so much as to appear normal, though fortunately this is uncommon. To reflect the importance of avoiding false reassurance from home kit results, the American Academy of Sleep Medicine

---

d See chapter 17 for more on sleep perception.

practice guidelines state that when home kits turn up negative for sleep apnea, this should be confirmed with follow-up testing in a sleep lab.[58] In 2017 we conducted a study to estimate how likely these underestimations were, based on a large population of adults who'd had in-lab testing done in our center, and we found that clinically important degrees of underestimation could have occurred in 20 percent of cases.[63] The problem was that we didn't find very useful clues to predict who was at risk for under-estimation.

The bottom line is that when sleep apnea is strongly suspected but the home test returns normal results, we may not know exactly why the sleep apnea might have been underestimated on that particular night for that particular person, so the safest bet is to get confirmation with additional testing. Having a sleep test done in the lab instead of at home does not entirely protect us from these issues. Some people don't spend much time sleeping on their back during a lab test, and in those cases, sleep apnea severity can be underestimated if the problem is happening mainly in the supine position. The main advantage of the lab with respect to these limitations is that the measurements are comprehensive, and the more information we have, the better we can interpret any given night of sleep. For example, because position is always monitored in a lab test (but is not the case for all home tests), we would not be easily tricked by a case of sleep apnea that depended on sleeping position during a night in the sleep lab.

What if a result of normal breathing from the home test is true, meaning there really is no sleep apnea present? There are two main paths to consider in this case, both of which could be confirmed by an in-lab test, as mentioned above. First, we could consider other sleep problems that home sleep apnea kits do not detect.[e] Second, the diagnosis could be what is called primary snoring, which means that the airway is obstructed just enough to cause the sounds and vibration of snoring but not quite enough to meet the criteria needed to diagnose sleep apnea. Snoring can be bothersome to the bed partner and family members, or it can lead to dry mouth or other symptoms. If the snoring is related to nasal congestion, then treatment can be considered with over-the-counter or even prescription medications to alleviate the congestion. Sometimes various anatomical problems are involved, such as a deviated nasal septum, an enlargement of the nasal turbinates (structures on either side of the septum), or the presence of nasal polyps. These anatomical problems can be

---

e See chapter 16 for more on periodic limb movements of sleep, and chapter 7 for other causes of sleepiness.

evaluated by an ear-nose-and-throat (ENT) surgeon for possible treatment options. Other nonsurgical treatment options include losing weight, reducing alcohol consumption (especially near bedtime), avoiding sleeping on the back, or treating acid reflux, each of which could contribute to the snoring.

If the home test is positive for sleep apnea, what's next?

Just as we should consider the different ways to interpret a negative home test result, we should do the same when the home kit turns up positive for sleep apnea. In particular, the level of severity can be an important motivator for pursuing treatment, and can even predict the response to treatment. The most commonly used mask treatment, and still considered the gold-standard choice for therapy, is continuous positive airway pressure, or CPAP.[f] This treatment path can be attempted for any severity of obstructive sleep apnea. The level of air pressure needed to treat sleep apnea with CPAP can vary tremendously from case to case, and the traditional standard for evaluating the appropriate pressure settings is to perform a CPAP adjustment night in a sleep lab, which is called a titration study. Alternatively, CPAP therapy can be started in the home without first coming to the sleep lab for a titration. This at-home path to treatment uses an automatically adjusting CPAP machine, or auto-PAP (also called APAP), which can vary the pressure levels during the night as it detects more or fewer breathing events, such as may occur with changes in body position or sleep stage. All modern positive airway machines, whether continuous or adjusting, capture important information to make sure the treatment is working as expected.[g]

Despite the status of CPAP as the gold-standard therapy for obstructive sleep apnea, it's not for everyone, and many patients are interested in alternatives.[h] Many factors, including patient preference, go into the decision of alternatives to CPAP. Even the information gleaned from a trial of CPAP can be helpful for choosing among the alternatives. For example, cases of sleep apnea that were treatable with low pressures of CPAP have more success with alternatives to CPAP. It is as if the low pressures were a signal to us that the person's airway was easy to keep open. A treatment called Provent nasal valves provides the equivalent of low-pressure CPAP, so knowing that a person's breathing has normalized with low pressures of CPAP is useful information, even if she

---

f See chapters 10 and 11 for more on the various options available for sleep apnea treatment.

g See chapter 10 for more on the usefulness of machine-captured data.

h See chapter 11 for alternatives to CPAP for treating sleep apnea.

cannot tolerate the CPAP mask itself, because this information predicts the effectiveness of Provent. Similar predictions have been made for the effectiveness of dental appliances, which work best in cases of sleep apnea that improved with low CPAP pressures.

Dental appliance effectiveness also depends on the severity of sleep apnea—which gets back to the question of how accurately the severity was determined by a home testing kit if dental appliance therapy is being considered. The most convincing data from clinical research studies is that dental appliances are most likely to work for the treatment of mild to moderate cases of obstructive sleep apnea. Some studies suggest that dental appliances can be effective even with cases of severe sleep apnea. Just as the tolerability and effectiveness of CPAP differs from case to case (which we'll discuss in chapters 10 and 11), so it is with the alternatives to CPAP. Dental appliance therapy and Provent can be combined with other treatments, such as position therapy or weight loss, to increase the effectiveness for improving sleep apnea. Surgical approaches are invasive and carry some risks, so in general, it might be more challenging to argue the benefits of surgery for mild cases of sleep apnea compared to a moderate or severe case.[i]

The change in sleep apnea severity according to body position is by far the best example of a diagnostic detail that helps inform treatment options. That position matters for sleep breathing has long been recognized; in fact, an entire textbook is devoted to the topic.[64] For a subset of sleep apnea cases, the obstructions only occur while sleeping on the back (the supine position), while breathing normalizes when sleeping on the side (left or right position). Such cases of position-dependence, which make up about one-third of all sleep apnea cases, can in principle be treated solely with position therapy, meaning avoidance of the supine body position. The principle of position therapy may not translate, however, into effective avoidance of the supine position in real-world practice. The consumer devices used for position therapy don't currently track body position, so we can't ensure that they are working as planned night after night. Some of these devices can move around during sleep and don't completely prevent lying on the back.[65] We should not assume it is enough to just ask people to avoid their backs (and then ask them how it's going), because body position can change in sleep without our awareness. One device, which is available by prescription, contains a position-tracking sensor and uses vibrations to alert users whenever they happen to roll onto their back during sleep.[66]

---

i See chapter 11 for more information about alternatives to CPAP.

As with any diagnostic test, we need to be mindful of placing the results in context. When test results agree with our expectations, things are more straightforward. If we strongly suspected sleep apnea based on someone's sleep story, and the home testing data confirms sleep apnea, then the information streams are aligned. But when the test results are unexpected, that's when we need to be careful, especially when a negative result occurs in someone strongly suspected of having sleep apnea, since this could be a false negative result. This well-recognized risk of home testing is why the clinical guidelines suggest that negative home tests for sleep apnea should be followed by an overnight test in a sleep lab for confirmation.[58]

CHAPTER 10

I wear a mask for sleep apnea. How do I know if it's working?

What information can we glean from the CPAP machine?

The CPAP machine stores various kinds of potentially useful information. The most basic information is the usage patterns, sometimes called compliance or adherence data. Insurance companies may require a certain minimum amount of usage to maintain coverage of the equipment—typically the threshold being at least four hours per night on at least 70 percent of nights. The machines also contain sensors for detecting air leakage and airflow patterns. Too much air leakage suggests that the mask is not fitting well onto the face, where it has to make a good seal against the skin. The airflow sensing allows the machine to detect interruptions in breathing, which is reported as an index of events per hour, similar to the apnea-hypopnea index (AHI) that's scored during a typical overnight sleep test. Higher values indicate that the machine is detecting interruptions in breathing despite wearing the mask, which suggests the CPAP treatment is not working optimally.

What if someone who uses CPAP feels better. Is that enough?

That's a great question—and while we'd like to celebrate symptom improvement with CPAP, it might not be enough for certain people with sleep apnea. We saw in chapter 8 how the symptoms of sleep apnea and the measurement of sleep apnea don't always correlate tightly. Just as this potential disconnect is important when thinking about the diagnosis of sleep apnea, it is also important when thinking about treatment response. In particular, we need to think about whether feeling better means that the sleep apnea is completely treated. In other words, could partial (but incomplete) improvement of sleep apnea be enough to feel great? If so, then someone who feels great after starting CPAP might still need some treatment adjustments. It would be easy to simply ask about symptoms and leave it at that. Consider a concrete example of when sleep symptoms might not match up with sleep measurements.[a] Let's say someone had severe sleep apnea with an AHI of 50 events per hour, and that number reduced to an AHI of 15 while he was wearing the CPAP mask. He might feel terrific because of this level of improvement. The residual sleep apnea level of 15 is still in the moderate range, however, and we would prefer to have the AHI be even lower—ideally less than 5. In that case, if we just went by the feeling of improvement, then we'd miss an opportunity to improve his sleep.

The question then becomes: How can we know how worried we should be? We may have a few clues from the CPAP machine which stores data about how well the machine is working. If that data indicates ongoing sleep apnea events, despite wearing the mask, this is our main clue that some adjustment is still necessary. We might worry more with certain medical problems like heart disease, or with medications like opiate painkillers, which can make sleep apnea more difficult to control.

Subtle clues could also prompt us to take a closer look at how well the CPAP is working. If changes in behavior or health (or effectiveness of CPAP!) occur very gradually over a long time frame, then the effect on our sleep might be too subtle to realize. For example, one clue could be gradually increasing caffeine usage, which might be related to gradually worsening sleep quality. Any number of possibilities might occur, from gradually reducing our responsibilities at work to allowing more and more sleeping in on the weekends. Gradual changes might not be easy to connect with sleep, especially if we could chalk them up to other explanations such as stress or a change in mood.

What happens when people with sleep apnea sleep without their CPAP machines?

Another key question! Even for those patients who agree to CPAP treatment and use it regularly, the average patient does not wear it 100 percent of the time he or she is sleeping. While there is ongoing debate about how much CPAP use is "enough," the field generally considers compliance to be defined as at least four hours per night on at least 70 percent of nights. This threshold is often applied in clinical practice (such

---

a See chapter 17 for more on sleep perception.

as for insurance coverage) as well as in most research trials for defining treatment success.

But if we look at bit closer at the numbers, we face an interesting problem: for someone who sleeps eight hours per night, this usage threshold represents only 35 percent of her time asleep. That leaves the majority of sleep happening without the mask. In clinical practice, it is not common to measure what happens when you sleep without the mask, so the honest answer is that we don't really know what happens when people with sleep apnea sleep without their CPAP machines. But you might guess that our concern is that the sleep apnea comes right back. From research studies, it seems that in at least half of patients who use CPAP, the sleep apnea returns to the untreated, or baseline, severity of sleep apnea when sleeping without the CPAP mask. In other patients, the sleep apnea doesn't seem to return right away when sleeping without CPAP, but rather it comes back gradually over a few nights. It is as if there is some lingering benefit of CPAP even from partial use, in these lucky folks.

You might think a patient would feel the difference, depending on which of those two possibilities, the rapid versus delayed return of sleep apnea, was actually happening. For some this is indeed the case, and they feel noticeably worse if they don't wear the mask the whole night or if they skip a night. Others might not notice much of a difference, and that makes it tricky to guess what's happening because of the same kind of disconnect of symptoms and measurements we've been talking about. More and more researchers are suggesting that we can use special devices to make these kinds of measurements (i.e., to look at breathing across the whole night) to determine the true effectiveness of CPAP treatment for sleep apnea in the real-world situation of partial use.[67,68] But until measurements become standard clinical practice, we will remain, well, in the dark about this question. Even without measuring directly, can make a guestimate according to how many hours a person sleeps with versus without CPAP on average, and assume that the sleep apnea comes back any time sleep happens without the mask. We've termed this approach "apnea burden", and estimates can be made with our free online calculator (www.apneaburden.com), ideally in discussion with a treating physician to help interpret the numbers.

What if someone with sleep apnea doesn't feel better with CPAP treatment?

This can happen in two main situations. One is when the person was already feeling pretty good before starting CPAP (that is to say, they had a disconnect between symptoms and measurements), and another is when the person actually did have symptoms of sleepiness or other problems but did not get better even after starting CPAP treatment. In the first case, where the patient felt fine before starting CPAP, then we would focus on the machine numbers as our main source of information about how effective the treatment was. In some cases, we could also track some other aspect of the person's health: let's say the patient had high blood pressure, then we might look for better control after starting CPAP—either lower values or lower doses of medication needed to control the blood pressure. Back to the second case: if the person had sleepiness or other problems but did not improve on CPAP, then we would want to think through some of the most common possibilities, which we will do now.

Mask: Getting the headgear right is a crucial step in successful CPAP treatment. The mask and straps should be comfortable, and the mask should not leak. If either leak or discomfort occurs, it can disturb sleep quality directly. And if air is leaking from the mask not fitting well on the face, that could be more than just annoying, it could also mean that not enough air is getting where we need it: into the airway to treat the sleep apnea. Having a mask-fitting session with a sleep technologist or respiratory therapist can be helpful.

Pressure: The level of air pressure the CPAP machine is blowing can be either too high or too low, and both can cause problems with proper treatment of sleep apnea. The pressure settings can be determined by an overnight test in the lab, but in some cases, the ideal pressures are not obvious. For example, if the patient happened to change body positions during sleep, and the test did not record any time in the combination of supine body position (on the back) and REM sleep—the most vulnerable situation for many sleep apnea patients—then the ideal pressure remains uncertain. Higher pressures may be needed during this vulnerable combination of supine-REM sleep. However, sometimes the CPAP pressure used is too high and can directly disturb sleep, and high pressures can even cause breathing to become unstable, a situation called complex apnea.[b] Another way to make the pressure feel more comfortable is to use a related kind of machine, called BiPAP or BPAP, where the "B" stands for bi-level (two-level) pressure. These machines are smart enough to know whether you are inhaling or exhaling, and give more pressure during the inhale (to match your effort), and less pressure as you exhale. BiPAP is also useful for patients who have low oxygen levels independently from sleep apnea, such as from emphysema or obesity, which is sometimes called hypoventilation.

---

b See chapter 11 for more on complex apnea.

Auto-PAP: An important advance in CPAP therapy was replacing the "C" in the acronym, which stands for continuous, with the feature of automatic adjustability of the pressure. These automatically adjusting machines are called auto-PAP, or APAP, and are designed to increase or decrease pressure depending on how the person's breathing changes throughout the night sleep. For patients who need very different pressures in REM versus non-REM sleep, or in supine versus non-supine body position, an auto-PAP can feel more comfortable than having a constant high pressure all through the night. On the other hand, sometimes the changing pressures from an auto-PAP can themselves disturb sleep and make it feel like too much (or too little) air is blowing. A simple solution in that case is either to change the range of pressures the machine can use, or to go back to the "C" mode (i.e., CPAP), choosing a middle-of-the-road pressure as a compromise to the auto-PAP range of pressures.

The last resort: We know that some people with sleep apnea have persistent sleepiness even after starting CPAP therapy and using it regularly, and none of the issues we discussed earlier in the chapter could explain the lack of symptom improvement. Some patients consider treating this ongoing sleepiness with a "countermeasure." This could mean adding some extra sleep, such as through napping, for those who have the time to do so and find benefits from napping. Or this could mean using caffeine, for those who feel an increase in energy from caffeine and don't suffer side effects or have other medical reasons to avoid caffeine. If people have no treatable reason for their sleepiness, and naps or caffeine are not viable options, then sometimes they try prescription stimulant medications. What we want to avoid is coming to this last-resort stage of medication before ruling out other possible causes (like thyroid problems, or perhaps depression), and making sure CPAP is working well. Stimulants have potential adverse effects on blood pressure and heart rhythm, as may occur with untreated or incompletely treated sleep apnea, so we need to be doubly careful with their use.

CHAPTER 11

I have sleep apnea, but I can't wear that mask. What else is there?

Isn't CPAP the gold standard treatment?

Yes, CPAP is considered the gold-standard therapy to treat obstructive sleep apnea by keeping the airway open during sleep. Of all the treatments for sleep apnea, our field has the most experience with CPAP treatment. Some patients with sleep apnea are fortunate and take to the mask right away and sleep with it regularly. Unfortunately, many patients with sleep apnea are not so lucky, and just cannot get over their struggles to adapt to it. Overall, approximately half of sleep apnea patients who initially try to use CPAP as their treatment will keep doing so in the long run. That's not a great success rate, but the point is, if you can't seem to make the mask work, you're not alone!

How can we help those who are struggling to wear a CPAP mask?

Before we talk through alternatives to CPAP, let's first review some ideas to help make CPAP workable. Many potential obstacles exist, but luckily, patients who are motivated to keep trying also have many potential solutions. Sometimes, just knowing that options are available is itself a motivating factor, and I always tell patients that we can troubleshoot many bumps on the road so they'll know what to expect. One of the most annoying problems with the mask is being woken up by air rushing out around the mask. Reducing or eliminating leakage can often be accomplished with a mask-fitting session. Even without leaking, the headgear itself can be bothersome, sweaty, or not maintain position over the course of a night of sleep. Although admittedly a trial-and-error process, this can often be improved with different styles of masks or accessories to reduce pressure points or other aspects of discomfort. The most common solutions to dry mouth (a common complaint) are to increase the humidification settings and to change from a nasal mask to a full face mask that covers the mouth and nose. Adding a chin strap can help if a nasal mask is preferred but mouth opening is occurring during sleep. If dryness still persists, sometimes insulating the CPAP tubing can help, especially if the bedroom is kept very cool, which can cause the humidity to condense within the hose before it reaches the mask. Nasal congestion is the enemy of every CPAP user; this can lead to mouth opening and often requires using higher CPAP pressures (which leads to more dryness and intolerance). Treatments range from saline sprays to decongestant medications and even surgical options for the tough cases, through consultation with an ENT surgeon. High CPAP pressures for any reason can make it hard to tolerate the mask, whether because of leakage or because the straps need to be tightened too much to prevent the leaking. Techniques to allow lower CPAP pressures to be effective include reduced leakage, improved nasal congestion, weight loss, and sleeping on one's side instead of on one's back (more on this important topic later in this chapter).

For some people, the amount of pressure needed to keep the airway from becoming obstructed during sleep differ throughout the night. For example, some people need higher pressures during REM sleep or while they are sleeping on their back. Auto-PAP machines (which we also mentioned in chapter 10) can be useful in such cases, as they can increase pressure to react to breathing obstructions if they worsen during the night, such as from sleeping on your back or entering REM sleep.

What is complex sleep apnea?

For a small portion of sleep apnea patients, more than just obstruction of the airway is causing interrupted breathing during sleep. Sometimes the nerve reflexes that control breathing while we sleep misbehave, which results in pauses in breathing even without obstruction. Unlike obstructive sleep apnea events, in this case the airway is open but there is no effort being made to breathe. This kind of sleep apnea is termed "central sleep apnea" to refer to the nervous system's involvement. For some people, we find this problem at the time of diagnosis, while others develop this problem only after starting CPAP, in which case it is usually termed either "complex sleep apnea" or "treatment-evoked central apnea." Complex sleep apnea is more common with high CPAP pressures and with two-level pressure (called bilevel-PAP or BPAP). Certain medical problems such as heart failure, and certain medications such as opiate pain-killers, have also been linked to increased risk of central and complex sleep apnea.

People with central or complex sleep apnea may have a difficult time tolerating CPAP or BiPAP, sometimes described as feeling either air hunger or inability to breathe comfortably. These sensations can also happen if a person is claustrophobic or if the pressures are simply set too high, so it's important to combine this information with other clues, such as breathing patterns during the in-lab titration night, or from data downloaded from the machine. If we observe central apnea from these data sources, this supports the conclusion that the poor tolerance of CPAP or BiPAP is due to complex apnea. Treatment with a different kind of machine, called adaptive servoventilation (ASV for short), can help solve this problem by adjusting how much air the machine blows according to your breath-by-breath patterns. ASV is different than autoPAP (which we discussed in chapter 10) in that the machine's algorithm is reacting to breathing patterns in a more detailed way. While the machine can be very helpful for many patients, there is one group that requires extra caution (that we mentioned way back in chapter 1!): people with advanced heart failure and central apnea, who should not use ASV because of risks detected in a recent clinical trial.

Alternatives to CPAP

Despite the best efforts of patients and their providers, wearing a CPAP mask at night is simply not in the cards for some people. In this case, we can consider alternative treatment options for sleep apnea.

Weight loss: For some patients, being overweight is the main reason they have sleep apnea in the first place. Although weight is a common risk factor, it can be hard to predict which patients will see their sleep apnea melt away as the pounds melt away. It is likely that some improvement in sleep apnea will occur with weight loss, but individual responses will vary. For this reason, it's important to repeat measurements of sleep apnea after major weight loss (at least 10 or 20 percent of body weight) to see how much improvement has occurred. Achieving weight loss is admittedly easier said than done, but the benefits would likely extend beyond improvement of sleep apnea, as many other health problems are linked to obesity.

Provent nasal valves: These are small adhesive valves that stick on each nostril for single-night use. The valves provide resistance to exhaled breath so that some of the air pressure gets backed up into the airway to keep it open during sleep. The valves provide a relatively low amount of back pressure, equivalent to a CPAP level of approximately 5 to 7. Because it is important to keep the mouth closed and only to breathe through the nose with this therapy, some people may need to wear a chin strap simultaneously with the valves to help keep their mouths closed during sleep.

Position therapy: For many patients with sleep apnea, sleeping on their back is worse for their breathing compared to sleeping on their side. They might notice this themselves, or their bed partner may notice because the person's snoring is louder when lying on the back. Overall, about half of patients with sleep apnea will have some degree of worsening while sleeping on their back. The most important piece of this body-position story is that for a subset of these patients, the sleep apnea *only* occurs when they are on their back—while their breathing is normal when they sleep on their side. We call this "supine-isolated sleep apnea." That subset can be managed, in theory, with position therapy to avoid sleeping on the back. This can be done with wedge pillows, or with belts that have "bumpers" at the back to make it uncomfortable if you roll onto your back. These are available as consumer products and do not require a prescription from a doctor, but if you are considering one of these for sleep apnea, it is best done through discussion with your doctor. A prescription device is available, which is a neck collar that uses vibration as an alert to shift position whenever a person rolls onto their back.[66]

Even if the sleep apnea doesn't completely vanish when people sleep on their side, we can often use body-position therapy in combination with another treatment option. This approach is based on the idea that it is easier to keep the airway open when people sleep on their side, whether using a CPAP mask or Provent valves or a dental appliance (coming up next).

Dental appliances: The idea behind these devices (also known as oral appliances) is that pulling the lower jaw forward during sleep will open up the airway and reduce sleep apnea. Dentists who specialize in these appliances will make a custom-fitting device after assessing a person's teeth, jaw structure, and musculature in order to plan the best strategy. Most devices can be adjusted to strike a balance between patient comfort and tolerance versus moving the jaw forward enough to open the airway and reduce or eliminate the sleep apnea. The best evidence is for using dental appliances to treat sleep apnea in the mild to moderate range of severity.[69] However, they can be considered in patients with severe sleep apnea as well, especially if they did not tolerate CPAP. Some studies have suggested that younger and less obese patients are more likely to experience success with dental appliances in treating their sleep apnea.

Palate surgery: This surgical procedure, which requires general anesthesia, involves removing some of the soft palate, including the uvula (that dangly thing at the back of the throat). In doing so, the airway becomes more open, and snoring is often reduced. The sleep apnea is not always improved by this surgery, however, with about half of patients still having persistent sleep apnea levels. The Ear, Nose, and Throat (ENT) surgeons who perform this kind of surgery will examine the airway, often with a fiber-optic scope, to make a better prediction about the chances of success.

Jaw-advancement surgery: This kind of surgery is much more involved than palate surgery, and the recovery time is much longer—but the advantage is that the success rate is also much higher. It is known as maxillomandibular advancement, to reflect the process of cutting the bones of the upper jaw (maxilla) and lower jaw (mandible), and using plates and screws to re-position the bones more forward to open the airway and reduce sleep apnea. The oral surgeons who specialize in this procedure will perform detailed examination and x-rays to plan the surgery and to make better predictions about success.

Tongue stimulator: This procedure involves implanting a device similar to a pacemaker (a small computer) just under the skin of the upper chest. The device senses when you are breathing, and with every inhalation it stimulates a nerve in the neck called the hypoglossal nerve that moves the tongue forward. Because the tongue can obstruct the airway during sleep, this stimulation can improve sleep apnea by keeping the tongue in a more forward position so it is out of the way from blocking the airway. The procedure was approved recently in 2014 after two decades of development, with the most recent clinical trials using a fiber-optic view of the airway during anesthesia to predict success: if the tongue is visualized to be the main source of obstruction during drug-induced sleep, then this visualization increases the chances of success of the stimulator reducing or curing the sleep apnea.

CHAPTER 12

I have trouble falling asleep

The experience of insomnia

t seems like an age-old battle: you end the day and are looking forward to the quiet respite of sleep, but it just won't happen. And while the reasons for this are as personal as there are people with this struggle, thinking through a few common categories can help prioritize the steps to combat this problem. In this chapter, we'll talk through the categories of *brain*, *body*, *bedroom*, and *behaviors*.[a]

Before we dive into the potential causes and treatment options, let's say hello to an elephant in the room. Insomnia is not about numbers—it's an experience, a very personal and qualitative sense of distress about sleep. This means that two people can both take thirty minutes to fall asleep, and only the one who is bothered by that delay is said to have insomnia. Actually any duration of sleep onset can qualify as insomnia if it is bothersome and occurs frequently enough. Although the diagnostic criteria do not mention any numbers to quantify what an abnormally long sleep onset period ought to be, how frequently the problem occurs is, strangely enough, very specific: at least 42 percent of the time (three or more nights per week). The priority of subjective experience over objective measurements is not simply an academic exercise; it is a reminder of just how personal the sleep experience is. It stands to reason that what is generally considered satisfactory treatment for insomnia would also be highly personal and qualitative. But when it comes to treatment response, the American Academy of Sleep Medicine provided guidelines for what is clinically meaningful in a 2017 publication about sleeping pills.[70] The consensus of that task force was that a ten-minute

---

a Some of this chapter will overlap with insomnia topics discussed in chapter 13. We'll also discuss sleep medications in that chapter.

improvement in sleep onset is considered clinically meaningful from taking a sleeping pill. Each person with insomnia who is reading this will react differently when thinking about whether ten minutes' improvement would be *personally* meaningful. The point is that we have another potential disconnect here, between experience and measurements, which will come up in the next chapter when we talk more about sleeping pills.

My brain won't turn off

My casual battleground metaphor at the opening to this chapter can itself be part of the problem for people with insomnia trouble: thinking of sleep onset as a battle, of wakefulness as the enemy, and tips and treatments as the ammunition transforms the bedroom into a kind of war zone. If each night comes with thoughts of sleep onset as combat—even when it feels severe enough to earn the metaphor—that introduces more hurdles in a vicious cycle!

Many people describe a feeling that they just can't turn off their brain. Maybe worried thoughts are intruding about today's unfinished tasks or tomorrow's growing to-do list. Maybe happy thoughts about positive things are distracting you from that transition into slumber. Maybe the quality and intensity of the mental ruminations are different from night to night. Maybe the mind isn't racing around at all, but is quietly keeping a vigil of alertness for reasons it seems unwilling to divulge.

For all the different descriptions of overactive brain we hear in the sleep clinic, I could mention many more types of advice for calming that brain back down. In fact, relaxation training is a core component of the standard treatment for chronic insomnia, known as cognitive behavioral therapy for insomnia, or CBT-I for short.[b] Ask a group of people what works best for them to relax, and the variety of answers will be dizzying. How to choose among the litany of apps, CDs, sound machines, meditations, and breathing exercises that are available? The short answer is that there is no single right answer. That's actually good news, because it means the options are plentiful, but that's bad news if you're the type to feel crippled by too many choices. Scented candles around a warm bath with wind chimes playing in the background might not be your cup of (decaf) tea, and that's fine. And if following a particular breathing sequence makes you feel competitive, or progressive muscle relaxations give you leg cramps, that's fine too, you have plenty of other options.

---

b See chapter 14 for more on CBT-I.

One way to think about relaxation techniques is to break them into categories and start with the category that seems most appealing, or to at least avoid categories that seem annoying or impractical. I like to break up the options into three categories: things you do, things you listen to, and things you think about. These may overlap, of course, and within each category are many flavors. Doing something could mean gentle stretching, light yoga, or taking a warm bath. Some people take a moment to write in a journal to put their thoughts somewhere else for the night. Listening can be done with or without headphones but ideally involves a timer to avoid inadvertently continuing the audio exposure throughout sleep. Are you the type to settle into a calm presleep Zen state from listening to an audio book or podcast, or do you prefer music or nature sounds? For the final category, taking the reins by modifying your own thoughts can be the most personal, and, for many, the most difficult thing to do. While the "doing" and "listening" categories place the focus externally, almost as if to distract you from your own thoughts, the focus becomes more about internal experiences with techniques such as meditation, prayer, and self-hypnosis.

Don't expect any of these to be "the best." Relaxation methods are not silver bullets that work for everyone. They are more like a roulette wheel. What wins for one person might be a dud for another, and what works for one person on one night might strike out for that person on another night. Having more than one relaxation method on your short list to draw from night to night may be the best bet.

Aligning body, bedroom, and behaviors

Sometimes it's not your mind that needs the calming, but rather the body that is getting in the way. Aches and pains are common barriers to sleep, and just as we each have different pain thresholds, we also have different vulnerabilities to pain competing with sleep. The firmness and type of mattress can affect pain, though this factor is also highly personal. Some people like the memory foam experience because it alleviates pain at certain pressure points on the body. Others may find the memory foam less comfortable than traditional mattresses because it is harder to easily change positions once you sink into it. If a new mattress is not financially feasible, then mattress toppers can simulate the memory foam experience with less of a cost commitment. Beds that are adjustable to provide elevation of the head or the foot are likewise a matter of personal experience as to their benefits. For example, elevating the head of the bed might help to alleviate acid reflux, but might also have the unintended consequence of increasing back pain. Sleeping on your side instead of your back might help reduce back pain (and also can reduce sleep apnea[c]) but might cause shoulder or neck pain. Pillows have even been designed to make side sleeping more comfortable from a neck and arm perspective.

What's in and around your bed can be as important as the bed itself. A bed partner who likes to read or watch TV can be just as problematic for sleep, especially if you're the kind of person who is bothered by earplugs or eye masks that might otherwise provide you some insulation from your partner's activities. And for the person who's already struggling with sleep onset, few things are worse than a bed partner who not only falls asleep within seconds of hitting the pillow but who also snores, thus creating the dual angst of jealousy and aggravation! In that case, unless you have really good earplugs or want to sleep in another room, have the bed partner read this book's chapters about sleep apnea. The bedroom environment can also be important. Common bedroom tips about keeping the room cool and dark can mean major improvements in sleep onset for some people, while others may find it hard to notice much difference. How cool, how dark, and how these changes are achieved (eye mask versus light blocking window shades, fan versus air conditioning) are very personal decisions (and environmental tricks can be difficult to align with a bed partner if they have a very different opinion).

For anyone who's concerned about falling asleep, it's very reasonable to look into the basic tips of sleep hygiene.[d] You might be surprised at how useful these tips are, but even if they don't pave the path to slumber smoothly enough, following sleep hygiene topics can still serve to minimize unnecessary obstacles before trying other techniques. Sleep hygiene extends to the choices we make even before we get ready for bed. Just as decisions that we make about the bedroom environment may face "competition" from a bed partner, decisions about the daytime may face competition of their own. We may consume caffeine for energy, but too much caffeine (or caffeine taken too late) could rob us of sleep. We may slip into a lovely nap, but if it's too long or too late in the day, then our nighttime sleep might suffer.

When sleep onset insomnia is a symptom of another sleep disorder

Two common sleep disorders can get in the way of initiating sleep. The first is more than just regular tossing and turning: a peculiar kind of restlessness in the legs, called

---

c See chapter 11 for a section on position therapy for sleep apnea.

d See chapter 6 for more on sleep hygiene.

restless legs syndrome, can start to act up at bedtime. The feelings are uncomfortable and can be hard to describe. Two important clues are that the symptoms come on or get worse at night and are improved or go away with movement or stretching. Some common causes include iron deficiency and certain medications. If this sounds like you, then chapter 16 is in your future. The second common problem stems from an inner clock called the circadian rhythm. While most of us have a circadian rhythm of sleep that is aligned with the time zone we live in, some folks have a delayed rhythm, as if they live in a time zone farther west than where they actually live. This is uncreatively known as "delayed sleep phase syndrome," the main problem of which is difficulty falling asleep. Figuring out whether a circadian rhythm problem is the cause of sleep-onset difficulties is pretty important because different recommendations apply, known as chronotherapy. If this sounds like you, then chapter 15 is in your future.

There is a third sleep disorder worth mentioning, even though it is not as common of a cause of sleep onset problems. We might not immediately think of problems such as sleep apnea causing difficulties falling asleep—after all, how can a problem that only happens in sleep be causing trouble for a person who has not yet fallen asleep to begin with? That seems like reasonable logic, except for the possibility that the person is actually sleeping during that early part of the night when he feels that sleep has not yet begun.[e] In that case, could it be that sleep problems such as sleep apnea are actually causing that feeling of sleep onset trouble? Sleep disturbance, including insomnia in the middle of the night, commonly occurs with sleep apnea, and we'll talk more about this in chapter 13. For some people with the combination of sleep apnea and insomnia, the perception of sleep duration improves once the sleep apnea is treated.[71]

---

e See chapter 17 for more on sleep perception.

CHAPTER 13

I have trouble staying asleep

Unpacking the causes of not sleeping through the night

Many of the same factors that potentially delay sleep onset at the start of the night can also lead to trouble throughout the night. In chapter 12, we explored the four categories of brain, body, bedroom, and behaviors, and these categories are just as important to consider for awakenings in the middle of the night as they are for getting to sleep in the first place. In this chapter we'll take a slightly deeper perspective to explore certain causes of awakening that are distinct from the various reasons that get in the way of returning to sleep once an awakening occurs. Think of the person who awakens to use the bathroom but then finds her mind racing with anxious thoughts once she tries to return to sleep. Or the person who wakes up because of an ache or pain but then finds his bed partner's snoring too disruptive to get back to sleep.

It can admittedly be difficult sometimes to distinguish whether the waking was solely caused by a bladder that needs relief or was for some other reason, and then we become aware of the full-bladder sensation. Similarly, with pain, it may be that a given amount of pain during sleep could be more or less likely to wake a person up depending on how light or deep her sleep happened to be at the time the pain was peaking. In other words, problems with sleep quality can give rise to awakenings during the night, whether or not the awakenings seem to also have their own independent (non-sleep) causes, such as pain, nocturia, acid reflux, hot flashes of menopause, or anxiety.

What about the specific problem of waking before my alarm goes off?

Medical writing about insomnia often divided it into three sub-categories: sleep onset or "early" insomnia (as in chapter 12), sleep maintenance or "middle" insomnia, and having the final awakening happen too early, which was given the unfortunate label of "terminal" insomnia. Early-morning awakening could simply be the last of several nighttime interruptions (and in that way, is just one piece of middle insomnia), or it could be the only interruption of the night, but the common theme is the inability to return to sleep before the alarm eventually goes off. Some people describe a light or half sleep during that final period if they remain in bed trying to sleep. Although some patients have told me that the early morning hours felt like the best sleep for them, from a biological standpoint sleep is typically the lightest at the end of a night (another interesting example of a disconnect between what a patient might say versus what a textbook might say). Some of the earliest studies on insomnia suggested that this pattern of early awakening was more common in those with depression, whereas difficulty falling asleep in the first place might be more common with anxiety. The clinical reality is not so clear-cut, where we see substantial overlap between insomnia patterns and psychiatric disorders. This is why it is important to consider psychiatric conditions when evaluating the potential contributors to insomnia (and why sleep is a crucial component of managing psychiatric disorders).

Although early-morning awakening can be associated with primary sleep disorders such as sleep apnea or periodic limb movements of sleep (PLMS), one sleep disorder is specifically associated with this insomnia pattern: a circadian rhythm problem called "advanced sleep phase syndrome." That problem is the flip side of "delayed sleep phase syndrome," which we discussed in chapter 12. When the circadian clock is not aligned to the current time zone but rather to one more eastward, this can cause awakening to occur earlier than intended. This misalignment can also cause people to go to bed earlier than they intend. People with this kind of sleep pattern are sometimes known as "morning lark" types. As in the case of delayed sleep phase syndrome, the treatment of advanced phase syndrome is through a strategy known as chronotherapy. Chronotherapy for advanced phase consists of two main parts: timed light exposure and gradual schedule change. For advanced sleep phase, the most important factor is the use of bright light in the evening, which pushes one's internal clock to later times. The schedule change involves moving the sleep zone (i.e., bedtime and wake time) later by thirty minutes or so every other day until the sleeper reaches the target zone.[a]

---

a See chapter 15 for more on circadian rhythm disorders and chronotherapy treatment.

Perception of sleep and wake (this is not a trick question)

But it sure sounds like a trick question.[b] I get that. Over the years at the sleep clinic and through lecturing about insomnia and perception, I've noticed that even asking about the difference between subjective and objective measurement of sleep can put people—patients and physicians alike—on the defensive. After all, what could be complicated about knowing if you are asleep or awake? Further, it's standard practice to diagnose and manage insomnia based on the subjective experience, without any need for testing in a sleep lab. I've even heard doctors argue that if the amount of sleep determined by the EEG recordings disagreed with the patient's estimate of sleep duration, then it must be that the EEG was wrong. These experiences made me appreciate that the conversations had inadvertently drifted into a realm of "right versus wrong." This seemingly confrontational implication could not be further from the intention of discussing that sleep has both subjective and objective features. It's not a matter of right or wrong. In past years, the distinction between subjective and objective sleep was a curiosity that neuroscience could not answer. In recent years, however, clinical research has revealed that the distinction between subjective and objective sleep duration is actually an important part of understanding insomnia as a disorder.

Once we start to think about how the distinction between subjective and objective sleep can be helpful for decision-making, we can see that insomnia involves much more than just sleep duration. But we should start with discussing the topic of sleep duration, since it is so central. In every sleep diary, every sleep survey, every sleep app, and every sleep clinic, in one form or another you'll hear the question, "How much sleep did you get?" It seems like it should be an easy question to answer.[c] For people who don't have sleep trouble, this question is nothing more than a subtraction problem (from the time to sleep to the time the alarm sounded) to figure out the duration of time they've spent asleep. For people who do have sleep trouble—those who generally don't sleep through the night—the question is not as straightforward as that, since they have to add up the blocks of sleep time, or subtract out the blocks of time they were awake, or use some other technique to summarize the total from several chunks of sleep throughout the night. Study after study shows a range of mismatch between the subjective experience and the objective measurement of sleep in the sleep laboratory.[77] For healthy adults without sleep complaints, the mismatch is "optimistic," in the sense that the subjective report of sleep duration is often greater than

---

b See chapter 17 for more on sleep perception.
c See chapter 3 for more on the topic of sleep duration.

the objective sleep duration. This is at least partially because people typically don't perceive or remember the brief minutes of wakefulness that may percolate through a normal night of sleep. For an adult with chronic insomnia, the mismatch is "pessimistic," in the sense that the subjective estimate is often lower than the amount of sleep measured objectively. As a further example to suggest that "optimism" and "pessimism" are appropriate terms here, one study compared subjective sleep durations each morning for several nights with an overall average (across all nights) requested after the study was completed.[27] The normal sleepers gave estimates even higher than the numerical averages of their each-morning estimates, while those with sleep problems gave even lower values than the average of their previous daily estimations. In other words, the normal sleepers were even more optimistic when thinking back over the week, while those with insomnia were even more pessimistic when thinking back over their week of sleep.

Although studies have documented mismatch between subjective and objective sleep duration for decades, only in the last five years has this topic become rooted more firmly in a health context. The driving force behind this shift is a large study from Pennsylvania State University, which showed that the health outcomes of adults with insomnia symptoms were determined almost entirely by the objective measurement of their sleep durations in the lab.[73] Following over one thousand people for over ten years, it turned out that the risks of high blood pressure, diabetes, depression, and even mortality were only elevated in those people who had the combination of insomnia symptoms and objective short sleep duration. Either one or the other in isolation was not associated with increased risk. This data suggests that perception of sleep duration is not just a curiosity for neuroscientists—objective sleep duration can be a marker of health risk, which means that it should be part of a conversation about risk-benefit discussions in the clinic, especially if people are considering sleeping pills to treat insomnia, which carry adverse effect risks (which we will discuss further later in this chapter).

How important is it to have a solid block of sleep at night?

Nearly every patient who has chronic insomnia, and probably many other people who are not diagnosed with insomnia, believe that sleep should occur in a solid block. This was not always the common belief. The historian A. Roger Ekirch has written extensively about the "two-sleep" pattern that was common until the early twentieth century, in his engaging book *At Day's Close: Night in Times Past.*[74] It was generally considered abnormal if one did *not* awaken midway through the night, having a period of active time that separated the night into first and second sleep periods. Putting aside potential cultural and societal reasons for the eventual shift to thinking that one block of sleep was better than two (which remains speculative, rather than a clear medical reason), we can ask an even more provocative question: Even on nights when we feel that sleep is happening in one solid block, will that perception be reflected in the brain waves on the EEG recordings in a sleep lab? Like most if not all mammals, human sleep is actually quite choppy when we measure it objectively. The EEG sensors can detect brief awakenings of between a few seconds and a few minutes in duration. The longer ones (a minute or more) may occur five to ten times in a given night without people perceiving or remembering them. The brief ones—those that are less than fifteen seconds or so—can happen ten to fifteen times *per hour of sleep*, and are even less likely to be noticed consciously. We can think of many phrases to describe such physiological observations, but "solid block" would not be high on the list.

How can we make sense of this when we think about insomnia? When we measure sleep objectively, people who differ only in the presence or absence of insomnia symptoms may have very similar-looking sleep duration and cycles measured in the sleep lab. In other words, we can't use the objective data from a sleep-lab recording to predict whether a person is bothered by insomnia symptoms or even remembers waking up during the night. That some people are bothered more by interruptions than others has long been a tough challenge for the field of sleep medicine: here we have a common problem of insomnia, and while we have modern advancements in sleep measurements, we cannot reliably answer the seemingly simple question of what makes sleep feel good or bad from case to case.[75] Perhaps this is not as surprising as it sounds, if we take a step back and think about the situation for sleep apnea, an arguably dramatic form of sleep disturbance, and we can't reliably predict who will feel sleepy (or not) for any given severity of that disease.[d]

Let's get back to real-world decision-making. Even if we can't make much sense of single nights of sleep recordings in terms of perception of sleep or severity of insomnia symptoms, we can still take a big-picture view of how sleep perception can guide us in practice. We might respond to new or worsening changes in sleep-wake patterns over time to help shape how worried we should be. New or more troubling interruptions in sleep, even if "just" by subjective perception, could be clues about underlying sleep disturbances. This touches upon a topic we mentioned earlier in the chapter:

---

d See chapter 8 for more on symptoms, and lack thereof, in cases of sleep apnea.

the awakening could be caused by something else (for example, a primary sleep disturbance like sleep apnea), and if so, the goal should be to address the root cause rather than focusing on the awakening itself without regard to cause. If the focus is too much on the interruption *per se*, then any decisions people make for treatment might be geared only toward eliminating awakenings, perhaps through medications, like placing a band-aid without addressing the root cause. In other words, we don't want to jump directly to "medicate" the awakening without understanding the potential causes of that awakening. This might seem obvious, and if so—great! But how to look for root causes might not be obvious, especially for people who might not experience any hints about the potential causes, so it might seem like the awakenings are for no particular reason.

Putting this all together, we can strike a balance between thinking that a solid sleep block is critical for healthy sleep and thinking that if interruptions are really so common, then there's no need to worry about them. How bothersome awakenings can be, this is a highly personal topic. But this is not just a philosophical question. Being bothered can translate into physiological arousal—akin to adrenaline release—and we don't need to debate whether that's going to help or hurt the experience of insomnia. Some of the most important strategies to improve sleep target the way in which we think about our own sleep. How we think about our own sleep is not just something "in your head", it has very real physiological implications. That is precisely why cognitive strategies to improve sleep through changes in our own thinking can be at least as effective as sleeping medications acting through chemical processes.[e]

Other sleep disorders that can cause insomnia symptoms

We'll make a distinction here between insomnia as a symptom and insomnia as a disorder. For someone who suffers from insomnia symptoms, this distinction might not be so obvious—which is precisely why we'll now talk it through. Essentially, we consider insomnia a disorder in itself (also called primary insomnia) if there are no obvious causes or contributors. When other causes or contributors are present, we might rather refer to the situation as insomnia symptoms. We already mentioned in an earlier section of this chapter one such problem, stemming from the circadian rhythm, called advanced sleep phase syndrome, which can cause insomnia symptoms.

---

e See chapter 14 for more on alternatives to medication, especially cognitive behavioral therapy for insomnia.

Three other common sleep disorders can be associated with insomnia symptoms: sleep apnea, restless legs syndrome, and periodic limb movements of sleep. If the second and third of these three disorders sound similar, then you're right: in some ways they are. Chapter 16 takes a deeper dive into both. Restless legs syndrome can interfere with sleep at the beginning of the night (as noted in chapter 12), and it can also cause problems with awakening in the middle of the night. The key feature of restless legs is that people experience the symptoms while they're awake. In contrast, periodic limb movements happen during sleep, so people may or may not know they're happening—this is similar to how sleep apnea can occur without a person realizing it. These leg twitches can interrupt the normal cycling of sleep and increase someone's chances of waking up throughout the night. Unfortunately, researchers have not studied the importance of these leg twitches nearly as much as they have studied sleep apnea. As a result, it is not currently common clinical practice to seek diagnostic testing solely to look for periodic limb movements in those who have insomnia. If polysomnography testing is performed and leg twitches are found to be prominent, however, then that can help inform treatment options.[f]

The main sleep disorder that is often overlooked as an underlying factor in someone who experiences nighttime awakenings is sleep apnea. Maybe it's overlooked because we think of sleep apnea as causing the opposite problem—too much sleepiness. Maybe we can appreciate that sleep apnea could cause brief awakenings, but what about longer blocks of time spent awake—how can sleep apnea be the cause in those situations?

Let's think through the ways that sleep apnea could be playing a role, and when we might be more or less worried about it. Many research groups, including my own, have found a surprising overlap between sleep apnea and insomnia[45-48]. We often can't say for certain whether one causes the other, since both are common problems in adults. It could be purely chance that some people have both problems, and those unlucky folks are the ones who end up in sleep clinics, because it's double trouble for their sleep. Despite the uncertainty here, we can play out other interpretations and see where they lead us. If we don't at least think of the possibility of sleep apnea in an adult who has chronic insomnia, we take three potential risks. First, we may miss the chance to diagnose a treatable sleep disorder (sleep apnea) with health implications, even if it turns out after successful sleep apnea treatment that the insomnia symptoms did not improve indirectly from treating the sleep apnea. Second, the chances of

---

f See chapter 16 for more on treatment of periodic limb movements of sleep.

successful insomnia treatment with cognitive behavioral therapy for insomnia (CBT-I) might be reduced if sleep apnea is present and is contributing to the insomnia, since CBT-I does not treat the underlying sleep apnea. Third, and perhaps most concerning, the use of sleeping pills in anyone who has untreated sleep apnea introduces the potential risk of worsening the sleep apnea, especially with certain sedative medications. Even if someone's breathing is not worsened by a particular medication, the effectiveness of improving their insomnia symptoms might be fighting a similarly uphill battle, just like with the CBT-I example, due to the untreated sleep apnea.

To revisit the topic of needing to visit the bathroom at night, we can think through a list of potential causes to include an anatomical problem (such as bladder abnormalities, or an enlarged prostate in a male), or a behavioral factor (such as excess liquid intake near bedtime), or because of untreated sleep apnea. These are very different causes with different implications for diagnosis and treatment. The first two are more direct causes of nighttime urination, but each has different treatment options. In the case of sleep apnea, in contrast, it doesn't directly cause the need to urinate, but rather the repeated interruptions in breathing can keep people in lighter stages of sleep, such that they become more aware of their bladder fullness through the night. Despite this potential connection, we can't interpret getting up to use the bathroom as a reliable sign of sleep apnea, because there are many other potential reasons to do so. And we also can't assume that reducing nighttime bathroom trips is a sufficient motivation, by itself, to treat underlying sleep apnea. But that gets back to filling in the information to help the patient with chronic insomnia make decisions: If sleep apnea is present, then how severe is it? How much risk am I willing to take by not looking into the possibility of sleep apnea at all? To add another twist, it's well known that menopause comes with insomnia symptoms for many women, but it is less well known that menopause also carries increased risk of sleep apnea (in fact, the male predominance in sleep apnea risk only applies when comparing to females before menopause; after menopause, the risks are similar between the sexes).

How do sleeping pills help sleep?

The textbook answer to this question is that sleeping pills artificially produce sleepiness, thereby helping people fall asleep more quickly and stay asleep throughout the night. It may seem logical that, if sleep is important for health, and I can't seem to get enough sleep, even when I try to make the time and follow good sleep hygiene, then taking pills to increase my sleep duration should be beneficial to my health. Most sleeping pill research focuses on the subjective aspects of sleep: the perception of sleep-wake time and quality of life. But the assumption that improvements in those areas also translate into improved physical health has never been tested. When the occasional research study has measured objective sleep-wake times in addition to the subjective perception, the improvements have seemed quite modest. The average amount of extra sleep found in most of these studies is ten to twenty minutes. But the possibility of gaining ten to twenty minutes of extra sleep is hardly what brings people with chronic insomnia to seek the attention of medical professionals. Most people who try sleeping pills are hoping for much more improvement than that. They are hoping to get more than an extra ten to twenty minutes, or at least to feel like they're getting more than that.

In many cases, the subjective sense of extra sleep is much stronger, with estimates of one or two hours, even when the objective data is still less than thirty minutes more of sleep. That's not to say those subjective and objective aspects of sleep aren't important—they are, of course, central to what brings patients to seek medical care for insomnia in the first place. But there is a catch: we don't have good evidence that improved sleep (whether by subjective or objective measurements) translate into improved health for the person taking sleeping pills.

What are the risks of sleeping pills?

You don't need to be in clinical practice for long before you realize that patients differ in their perspectives on sleeping pills. I've heard patients explain their opinions about sleeping pills with everything from "I know someone who..." to "I read an article about" such and such treatments. These experiences fit into the patient perspective, just as physicians' experiences and their interpretations of the research on the topic fit into their perspectives. Some patients are against medication of any kind, while others assume without a second thought that anything they're prescribed for sleep will be safe and effective. Most people are somewhere in between.

The reported side effects of sleeping pills are extensive. They include effects on waking function the next day, long-term risks, drug-drug interactions, drug-alcohol interactions, and even effects on sleep quality (yes, you read that right, some sleeping pills can actually make sleep worse!). One of the most common concerns involves residual grogginess sneaking into the following day—what some describe as a hangover effect. One such next-day effect has drawn extra attention from the FDA, and rightly so: the residual effect of sedation lasting into the morning hours has been linked to increased motor vehicle accident risk. As a result, the FDA issued new warning labels in 2014 about the sleeping medication zolpidem,[76] (a common brand name being Ambien) including a lower recommended dose for women, since they may process the drug more slowly than men. The FDA more recently (in 2017) issued general guidelines for drug companies that test new medicines that could potentially impair driving.[77]

The risks that sleeping pills pose to sleep quality are also troubling, precisely because these effects might go unnoticed. Some sedatives can increase the risk or the severity of sleep apnea, for example, which can go undiagnosed in people with chronic insomnia. Some medications can make periodic limb movements (PLMS) worse, which can interfere with sleep quality. Because diagnostic testing is not required before (or after) people start using a sleeping pill, in many cases these potential changes to sleep quality remain unexplored, unless the patient is "lucky" enough to have symptoms that alert them to a problem after starting the sleeping medication. Other common concerns include a feeling of unsteadiness when getting out of bed in the middle of the night, which includes a risk of falls. When taken over the long term, even intermittently, the list of potential risks is long and includes everything from increased infections to elevated cancer risk, and even increased mortality.[78] Despite years of research to try to understand these risks, many uncertainties remain, which brings us back to the recurring theme of needing to place information in context for each individual to weigh the risks and benefits. Admittedly, this is especially challenging when the potential risks of long term medication use may be similar to the potential risks of chronic insomnia.

Treating insomnia: risks, benefits, and goals

We've touched on some of the root causes of nighttime awakenings. Identifying and modifying the root causes can go a long way toward improving sleep. This approach may not be a home run for everyone, but this is a key first step, if only to pave the way for subsequent efforts, whether they're sleep-hygiene tips (as discussed in chapter 6), medications (this chapter), or other drug-free approaches (chapter 14). This is all a lot to think about. As we've seen in this chapter, at least thinking through the options can help prioritize the steps toward getting better sleep that will make the most sense to each person, or at least that avoids stumbling into unnecessary risks.

The American Academy of Sleep Medicine recommendation is to limit prescription use to short term (perhaps a couple of weeks), but the reality is that many people use sleeping pills more regularly, making the risk-benefit balance efforts even more important. One way to summarize the goal of this balance, and to see how personalized this balance must be, is to ask a question: Do I feel sufficiently better taking a sleeping pill, compared to other treatments for insomnia, that taking it off-sets the potential risks? Since no research data to date has shown any physical health benefits from increasing sleep duration through chemical means, the "benefit" part of the balancing act focuses on quality of life, and that's about as personal as it gets. This is a delicate dance that applies to every kind of medication, not just sleeping pills, and this dance should end with us feeling confident that the benefits outweigh the risks.

To capture some of the major concerns about medications for insomnia, let's first consider a situation that I think we would all agree should be avoided. If someone takes a sleeping pill and then feels worse the next day, then we have a terrible risk-benefit balance. Even if she reports reaching her target amount of sleep (say, seven hours), if that doesn't translate into something—anything—about quality of life being bet-ter, then we are mixing up our priorities. This would be more like a sleep-at-all-costs approach, and the net effect could be that it does more harm than good. As we men-tioned earlier, the logic seems as if it should be this: if insomnia and sleep loss are associated with poor health outcomes, then cranking up the hours, even with the use of a pill, should reverse or prevent those risks. But unfortunately, the available research evidence does not support this logic. It's a major conundrum for the sleep field, and for patient-physician discussions of treatment options. If a therapy had no side effects or health risks, then this would be a simple discussion. But all pharmacological thera-pies (including herbals) have potential risks.[g]

Everyone who considers taking a sleeping pill should be able to look in the mirror and say, "My life is so much better with the pill than without that I'm willing to accept the risks of the treatment." But confirming that we feel better during the day is just the first step. Let's think of an analogy where a physician would say no to a treatment choice because of its known health risks: using alcohol to help us sleep. Some people might feel like they can fall asleep more easily after a drink or two—and they might even feel an overall subjective benefit of the drinks. If the subjective sleep experience is really the gold standard when it comes to insomnia, why don't sleep doctors support a choice for alcohol? Well, based on the risk-benefit balance we just talked through, we're essentially saying that the risks are too high, no matter how much better you may feel, for us to recommend alcohol for sleep (worse sleep quality, increased sleep apnea risk, and other health concerns with chronic use). Getting back to medications, we often have to strike this kind of balance but without having the benefit of objective

---

g See chapter 14 for more on herbals.

measurements of sleep, even though we know sleep quality may be worsened by some of these medications.

I admit that for the person struggling with insomnia for many years, it is no easy task weighing risks and benefits of sleep medication. Many factors have shaped patients' experiences with insomnia. Feeling like they've tried everything, fearing that they're helpless to improve, seeing every night as a battle, wondering why they can't just sleep like a normal person, being worried of health consequences from lack of sleep—these thoughts can build and dominate their experience and, in a vicious cycle, perpetuate the very problem they are desperate to treat.

Some people truly feel they cannot sleep (at all) without a sleeping pill. One way in which certain people arrive at this conclusion is that they have tried to stop taking the sleeping pills, and found that the insomnia immediately returned or even worsened. While at first glance this might seem to confirm that the pills were necessary, an alternative explanation is more likely. Especially for people who use a sleeping pill every night, stopping that usage can cause rebound insomnia, which is like a kind of withdrawal from the medication. Everyone varies in how much rebound insomnia might occur. Likewise, people vary in how long and how slowly their reduction in dosing should be in order to avoid rebound. Some patients don't take their sleeping pills every night, and so they may already have a sense of how much rebound will occur from their dosing experience. This can provide some important perspective when planning to reduce sleeping pill dosing among those who use medication nightly, through asking about what happens on nights when they went without their medication for any reason (whether on purpose or not).

Sometimes just the way people who struggle with chronic insomnia think about sleep can negatively affect sleep. Some in the clinical world have adopted the phrase "dysfunctional beliefs" to capture this paradox, which sounds unnecessarily harsh: that the very way we think about insomnia can make it worse. I've heard behavioral therapists describe this problem as needing to get out of one's own way, so to speak, on the path to treating insomnia. This can be particularly challenging, because some of the beliefs that the sleep medicine field considers dysfunctional may have their roots in information from our field that reaches the public. Let's take the recommendation for healthy adults to get seven to nine hours of sleep as an example. If patients interpret this recommendation too strictly and without context, some become too focused on achieving this duration. OK, maybe more than just some: it turns out that the number one item on the commonly used clinical tool the "Dysfunctional Beliefs and Attitudes about Sleep" scale is, you guessed it, "Need 8 hours of sleep."[79]

Regardless of what path we take toward improving sleep, it is important to think through the goals of therapy. Life seems to always be busier than we'd like, and we don't want to lose track of sleep patterns at the very time we need to track them—when we're making the effort to improve things! This means keeping tabs on what outcomes of treatment are most meaningful, and I will stress that this must include something about how waking life is better, rather than "just" something about sleep improving. This may sound obvious, but it is all too common to become over-focused on something about sleep, whether it's a certain number of hours of sleep, or a certain number of awakenings, or a certain time to fall asleep. Each of these sleep factors carries its own symptoms and frustrations, which will be different for each person. Sleep diaries and apps always include such features about the nighttime, but it's just as important to track what gets better about the day—and this is also highly personal.

Why is tracking the daytime waking experience so crucial? I can think of two reasons. First, looking at the daytime takes some of the pressure off of focusing on the nighttime. Nothing is more ironic than when our very efforts to improve "the numbers" of our sleep-focused diary entries cause anxiety about the numbers and perpetuate the insomnia. Whether you have, say, three versus two awakenings in a given night is less critical than whether any improvement about the night translated into something being better about the next day's experience. Second, if we're considering medications, we want to avoid focusing too much on the sleep diary numbers at the expense of daytime function. To provide a concrete example, we want to avoid the situation of taking a sleeping pill that eliminates awakenings and extends sleep duration but lacks the benefit of improving energy or quality of life the next day. For some people, the medication lingers into the next day, causing grogginess or fogginess, such that quality of life is actually worse even if the sleep diary values got better. Since long-term medication use has been associated with health risks (as we discussed earlier in this chapter), if we can't point to a personal benefit of something related to quality of life, then we find ourselves in a very shaky risk-benefit discussion. Admittedly, when multiple things are going on in our lives—with work and family stress, mental-health concerns, other medical problems, and the medications given to treat them—it can be hard to conclude how much better the day feels.[h] It's certainly easier to track whether something about sleep got better. Removing the worry about sleep might itself be an important goal, but it probably shouldn't be the only goal.

---

h See chapter 19 for more on self-discovery and diary tracking.

CHAPTER 14
Can anything besides medications help me sleep?

The gold standard: cognitive behavioral therapy

For more than ten years, the American Academy of Sleep Medicine has recognized the strong evidence that the gold-standard approach for chronic insomnia isn't a drug but rather cognitive behavioral therapy for insomnia, or CBT-I for short.[50,80] CBT-I is really a collection of techniques that are tailored to each individual over the course of several sessions of evaluations, skill building, and making effective changes to help sleep. It is much more than sleep hygiene, though as mentioned in chapter 6, such tips can be helpful building blocks. Some of the core components include using relaxation techniques, finding patterns in sleep diaries, and reversing negative thinking about sleep. One of the most interesting—and effective—components is known as sleep-restriction therapy. This approach is designed to reverse the tendency of people with insomnia to spend more and more time laying in bed, in an attempt to get some more sleep. This seemingly natural reaction to insomnia can actually make things worse and perpetuate the vicious cycle of insomnia. If a person repeatedly spends much longer times in bed, what sleep does occur is more likely to be fragmented and interrupted by time awake, which is the exact kind of problem we want to avoid. Sleep restriction is a temporary reduction in the time spent in bed, guided by the CBT-I program, to reverse this vicious cycle in a gentle and careful way.

Clinical research studies continue to support this approach, which is great news for patients looking for nondrug solutions for insomnia. And in case anyone thinks CBT-I is only for easy or mild cases, evidence from experiments comparing CBT-I directly to prescription sleeping pills shows the real muscle of this technique: the results are as good or even better than pills. For those who are already taking sleeping pills to treat insomnia, CBT-I can help with weaning their usage. For those who don't have the luxury of having a CBT-I specialist where they live, CBT-I has seen growth in clinically validated online options (examples include www.shuti.me, and www.sleepio.com).[81-84]

What about herbals and supplements for sleep?

It is certainly not uncommon for people with insomnia symptoms to try one or more of these kinds of remedies.[85,86] The two that have been studied most extensively are valerian root extract and melatonin,[87-89] the latter of which is a naturally occurring hormone. Another common over-the-counter solution is the use of a sedating anti-histamine like diphenhydramine, which is often an ingredient in "PM" formulations together with pain medicines (like ibuprofen). Unfortunately, the results of research studies that have used objective measures of sleep have not been encouraging for these remedies increasing sleep duration. As is the case with a few prescriptions, however, certain herbal remedies (such as valerian root) seemed to improve subjective reports of sleep,[90] even when the objective data showed little effect. Doctors tend to regard this kind of data with skepticism, especially because we lack careful safety assessments of herbal remedies that are not regulated by the FDA. One way to see the physician's perspective is to consider the kinds of debates we have within the field about the research trials that investigate prescriptions—across hundreds or even thousands of participants—and how hard it can be to understand the details and to agree on an interpretation of the results. By comparison, are we to hold a lower or softer standard for small-scale studies or single-person anecdotes? The history of medicine is full of examples where a common practice was found to be useless or even harmful once it was studied within formal clinical trials.[91]

But what about the perspective of the patient with chronic insomnia? You could argue that those people who actually experience chronic insomnia may not put the same premium on evidence-based standards as doctors do. For example, patients who used complementary and alternative therapies for their health concerns reported in a survey study that they would continue to do so, even if clinical trials showed that there was no effect of the treatment.[92]

I commonly hear about this or that news story claiming that some natural remedy is revolutionary, or guaranteed, or (playing to the attractiveness of conspiracy theories) that the remedy is the secret to sleep that the drug companies don't want you to know about. The hyperbole can be very creative, in part because these remedies are not subject to the same regulations as prescription drugs. This is very frustrating, as the expectations are set high, but the evidence to back up the claims is lacking. Still, the situation serves as a reminder of what kinds of information people with sleep trouble may encounter in the real world, whether or not they are consulting with a doctor or sleep specialist.

The American Academy of Sleep Medicine published updated guidelines in 2017 on sleeping pills, including over-the-counter pills such as melatonin and herbals.[70] The consensus was to recommend against the use of supplements and over-the-counter sedatives to treat insomnia (including melatonin, by the way), similar to the recommendation of the previous academy consensus statement from 2008.[50] The academy's rationale was based on the lack of data showing clear effects on improving sleep as well as uncertainties about safety. One major update in the 2017 guidelines was the recommendation against using the common medication trazodone for similar reasons. Trazodone is one of the most widely prescribed sleeping pills (even though it is "off label", that is, not FDA approved for insomnia), and the recommendation against its use is a reminder of the sometimes wide chasm between clinical practice and research evidence.

The academy recommendations are against herbals. How should we counsel patients?

This is where we really start to talk about medicine as an art form. One guiding principle is, of course, transparency: patients should be made aware of guidelines and whether a treatment under consideration is FDA approved or not. It's also important to consider if a risk is associated with *not* discussing treatments outside the FDA and practice guidelines, especially if a patient inquires about them. We sleep specialists are in a position not only to provide information about why certain recommendations are in place, but also to understand what is important to patients in terms of their treatment preferences and risk tolerance. Risk-benefit discussions can extend to herbals and over-the-counter agents, especially if the patient has expressed interest or is already trying these options. The conversations are quite similar, actually, as natural remedies also have potential risks,[93,94] even though some people may assume them to be safe simply because they're natural (many natural things are highly toxic!). One issue is the lack of regulation, which in one recent report led to concerns about product preparation and purity.[95] For patients who still wish to try natural remedies, several resources are available online to consult about possible adverse effects and drug-herbal interactions, product recalls, and other safety-related information, including:

- a liver toxicity database from the US National Library of Medicine for drugs and supplements (www.livertox.nih.gov);
- ConsumerLab.com's website on which brands have undergone independent testing (www.consumerlab.com);
- an FDA website for safety and product recalls, including food and herbals (www.fda.gov/safety/recalls).

We can have a similar kind of risk-benefit conversation about relaxation methods and other alternatives to help sleep, such as yoga, meditation, or acupuncture. The risks are different from something that is ingested, but we can still discuss them in a balance with cost and expected benefits. The medical evidence for these kinds of treatments to improve sleep is uncertain, but interest in the field remains strong. Further research may help us understand which therapies may work for which subtypes of insomnia as alternatives to drug therapy.[96] Some approaches, such as breathing-based relaxation methods, are particularly interesting, as we know that slow and controlled breathing calms the autonomic nervous system (known as the fight-or-flight, or adrenaline system), which is something that is thought to happen during normal non-REM sleep. Factors such as lowered heart rate and lowered blood pressure may figure into why these breathing exercises are calming. Whether people are trying hypnosis, breathing exercises, or acupuncture, my feeling is that the pressing question is whether they're gaining any benefits to their sleep experience, more so than knowing for certain why these things work. Knowing the answer to why would be like icing on the cake, but even if we don't know *why*, if we experience *that* it worked, then we have achieved the goal. This is certainly more so than the reverse situation: few people would find solace in an entire book about why a treatment should work if their personal experience was that it did not!

The tension between modern evidence standards and alternative remedies is also interesting from a pragmatic standpoint: is it feasible for evidence standards to be accomplished for herbal remedies for insomnia? Consider the vast number of herbal and alternative remedies that are currently available for insomnia: How much time and money would it take to obtain medical-grade testing for each them? For some people with sleep problems, waiting for better evidence to support herbal remedies is the sensible thing to do, even if, from a logistics perspective, this is unlikely to happen any time soon. For others, their risk-benefit perspective would allow them to explore this area even when it lacks good medical evidence. Either way, candid discussions of evidence and uncertainties, whether it refers to a prescription or an herbal, supports good decision-making. At the very least, we avoid the alternative that people don't discuss their sleep problems with a physician and make decisions based on incomplete or overly optimistic information curated outside of a medical context.

CHAPTER 15

Could I have a circadian rhythm problem?

The two clocks that drive sleep-wake rhythms

Many people are familiar with the idea of an inner clock keeping time for us, and even more so with the Nobel Prize in 2017 going to researchers in the field of circadian rhythms. Our inner clock sits in a very small area deep in the brain, so small that it cannot be seen even in modern brain scanners. The neurons in this area, the suprachiasmatic nucleus, are very sensitive to light detected by the eyes, which is conveyed to the clock area and results in the suppression of melatonin normally produced by the brain. Melatonin is the "darkness hormone," and for diurnal animals like us humans, night means sleep. Nocturnal animals like mice also have a melatonin rise at night, but in their context of being regularly awake during the night, melatonin (and darkness) does not mean sleep—another reminder that context matters!

What about the second clock? The brain uses a totally different system, one that is less well understood than the circadian clock, to keep track of time in a very different way. Whereas the circadian clock keeps track of time relative to the sun like a regular clock, the homeostat is a type of clock that keeps track of how long you have been awake or asleep recently. After a normal night of sleep, the homeostat starts ticking when you wake up and start your day. The longer you are awake, the more sleep "pressure" builds in this system, which translates into feeling more and more sleepy in preparation for subsequent bedtime. Say you're on a regular schedule of sleep from 11:00 p.m. to 6:00 a.m. As bedtime approaches, assuming you haven't traveled recently, both time-keeping systems, circadian and homeostat, agree that it's time for sleep. In contrast, someone who's pulling an all-nighter for school or work has both systems working against her, and fighting sleepiness can be challenging, to say the least. Caffeine is one of the most common countermeasures used to combat sleepiness—but caffeine only works through the homeostat by blocking some of that sleep pressure that's building up (by interfering with a chemical system called adenosine). Put another way, when you drink coffee, one of the reasons you find it energizing is that the homeostat thinks that you haven't been awake for as long as you actually have. Naps are another common countermeasure to combat sleepiness. Like caffeine, naps work against the sleep pressure sensed by the homeostat. But like caffeine, there is a potential downside: the longer the nap and the closer to bedtime it is, the less likely the homeostat will favor more sleep once bedtime actually arrives. This is why one of the sleep-hygiene recommendations for reducing insomnia is to avoid late or long naps.[a] This idea will also factor into jetlag, which we'll discuss at the end of this chapter.

What about screen time and blue light?

These two topics could not be more perfect for understanding the importance of context. But they often seem to be discussed out of context: we hear more and more that nighttime screen exposure, and especially light that is blue in color, is bad for sleep—period. Any questions? We could back up this concern by citing research studies showing that blue light is the color that most blocks the brain's production of the natural sleep chemical melatonin and that screen exposure before bedtime disrupts sleep continuity.[97,98] On the other hand, we could reasonably question whether the research studies apply in complex real-world settings.[99] After all, it doesn't take much light (of any color) to block melatonin production after sundown—and humans have had artificial light after sundown ever since humans gained control of fire, and obviously since the more recent inventions of electricity and light bulbs. Screen light in general is no more likely to suppress melatonin than most regular lamps, because the brightness of light matters (not just the color). In research studies, the sleep-wake experience is controlled in a very particular manner so as to isolate the experimental effects of light or screen time. In the real world, for most people, light exposure after sunset is a common occurrence and is but one wave in a sea of other variables that can affect sleep and alertness. This is what we call "noise" in the system, and it can be hard to decide how important any particular wave would be.

---

a See chapter 6 for more on sleep hygiene.

The complexity of the real world doesn't mean we ignore the issue of light and melatonin suppression. To strike a middle ground between living in fear of screens and brazenly sleeping every night with the TV on and phone in hand, we could help people think about placing this question in context. If TV or phone time is part of your wind-down routine (or reading and old-fashioned book with a bedside lamp, for that matter), and you're not having sleep trouble, it's hard to build a case to change this routine. But if you are having sleep trouble, especially with falling asleep in the first place, reducing screen time (for the light exposure, and the content exposure) is low-hanging fruit that might do some good. For those who just can't seem to shed their screen time, but they think it might be affecting their sleep, they can use a few tricks to help wean themselves away. Facing away from the screen, or trying an audio-only program, can be intermediate steps on the path to preserving the dim-light bedtime ritual. But even these things can cause people to become more alert (and less likely to sleep) based on the contents of what they're viewing or hearing, regardless of the light level.

Again, it's key to think about your own context to figure out what makes the most sense. What if having a two-hour wind-down time before bed, including dimming the lights and enforcing no screen time, does not seem practical for my life? What if that is my only time to catch up on family updates, or my only time to exercise, or any number of other sacrifices I would have to make of things that are important to me? What if my screen time is a meditation app that I find useful to calm my mind before bed? If I am only given the "rule" against screen time before bed, am I equipped to make an informed decision about how worried I should be? We can reconsider the situation as a trade-off. If someone uses a smartphone to calm down with a relaxation app, does the app work well enough to outweigh the risk of light exposure for a very sensitive person, or the tendency for some people to peek at news or email one last time on their phones?

On the topic of context, we should keep the bigger picture in mind when deciding to limit screen time. Think about regulating light and screen time in someone who uses caffeine or alcohol close to bedtime, or who has untreated sleep apnea, or pain-related sleep disturbance. Even if a person was sensitive to light, changes in screen exposure alone might have less of an impact in such situations with competing factors at play that could be interfering with sleep. Screen limits can still be part of a bigger-picture plan to optimize sleep, if those other obstacles are tackled concurrently. Considering our own context seems well worth the effort—informed choices are more likely to stick. The point is to figure out how to proceed (i.e., where to put your energy) by matching what is feasible, what feels reasonable, and what trade-offs you might have to make.[b]

Night owls and morning larks

We all know people who tend to drift away from society norms for sleep times in one direction or the other. We may have noticed our own tendencies might drift with age, or in different work or travel circumstances. Night-owl types feel more comfortable staying awake later at night, and they can sleep later in the morning. The reverse tendency, early to bed and early to rise, is true for morning-lark types (though sadly there is no science to support the ending to that adage, of early rhythms making us healthy, wealthy, or wise). Age may be the biggest factor to explain the variations: teens and younger adults are more likely to have night-owl tendencies, while morning-lark tendencies are more common among older adults.

For adults without symptoms and who are not bothered by their sleep timing in terms of health status, work needs, or personal life obligations, it is uncertain whether "treating" a night-owl or morning-lark so their sleep timing becomes more matched with the current time zone is necessary. The night-owl and morning-lark tendencies occur on a spectrum in terms of how bothersome or severe they are, as well as how modifiable these tendencies are by treatment with chronotherapy (more on what this is in a moment). Because of this variation, in order to make a diagnosis of delayed or advanced sleep phase syndrome, night-owl or morning-lark types need to feel a negative impact on their lives in some way, such as on work performance, sleepiness, or other health-related issues. Anchoring the thought process in such important context can then provide justification and motivation for pursuing treatment. A very risk-averse view might draw from research experiments and epidemiology studies of shift workers to make the argument that sleep is disrupted when it occurs at odds with the current time zone and that, over the long term, this misalignment can have a negative impact on health and well-being. A less risk-averse perspective is that many people seem to function well and maybe even enjoy their rhythm, even if it is very advanced or delayed compared to the average person. Whether such people decide to leave well enough alone requires, as always, a bit of context on a case-by-case basis.

One important aspect of decision-making is that some people with rhythm abnormalities seem as if they have insomnia when they seek medical attention. For

---

b See chapter 19 for more on self-discovery.

example, a night-owl type might describe his problem as "having trouble falling asleep." A typical example is the college student who was able to plan classes and social activities around their night-owl schedule, but then graduates and starts a job that requires him to wake up early. He might start trying to get to bed earlier than usual but find it challenging, perhaps even problematic enough to speak to a doctor about it. This situation can on the surface sound like "regular" insomnia, and it might even be associated with anxious nights and sluggish days because of insufficient sleep—also typical of insomnia. Likewise, a morning-lark type might find herself waking earlier than she would like and lingering in bed in the morning, frustrated at not being able to fall back asleep as long as she'd like to. If that situation were bothersome enough to seek medical attention, then she might describe her problem as having difficulty staying asleep. It is important to distinguish whether the problem is a circadian one, and thus it is best treated with chronotherapy. One major clue is that, when sleep is allowed to happen at the preferred timing (like the college student example above), there are no insomnia symptoms. Using medications such as sleeping pills would not be appropriate, because such pills do not fix the root cause, which is a circadian rhythm problem.

What is chronotherapy?

Chronotherapy consists of three categories (light exposure, melatonin dosing, and schedule shifting), and together they are used to gradually adjust a person's inner clock to be more aligned with his current time zone. Because the timing of each category of chronotherapy is crucial, we first need to make an estimate of where a person's clock is positioned relative to her home time zone. Why just an estimate? Because, surprisingly, we cannot directly measure the circadian rhythm in clinical practice, although some research methods are still being developed, such as detecting melatonin levels in the saliva as a clue about one's rhythm. The way to estimate people's natural timing is to map out what is actually happening with sleep and awake times in a diary and to ask about what timing they would prefer if they had no constraints of work or personal life. Often the night owls will drift into later sleep times on Friday and Saturday nights, thus sleeping later on Saturday and Sunday mornings, but then they have trouble again starting from Sunday night, when they try to get back to being aligned with work during the week. Some authors have termed this weekend-weekday jostling of sleep time "social jet lag," because it mimics the time zone shifts of air travel, and it is common among night-owl types.

Once a person's natural sleep zone is estimated, then chronotherapy can be planned out. The toughest part of chronotherapy to follow is the gradual shifting of the sleep zone over time—it takes a lot of discipline. A typical pace for doing this is about thirty to sixty minutes every other night. Let's say a person has a natural zone of 2:00 a.m. to 9:00 a.m. If her goal is to maintain seven hours of sleep but to target an earlier timing (say, from 11:00 p.m. to 6:00 a.m.), then it would take about two weeks to gradually move the sleep block three hours earlier at a pace of thirty minutes every other day. Melatonin can be added to help anchor the nighttime aspect of the rhythm. When used for this purpose, it is best to take melatonin about 2 or 2.5 hours before the planned bedtime, rather than at bedtime which would be too late to affect the circadian rhythm. That way, the timing of the melatonin level matches the more natural rise of melatonin that would occur at sundown were it not for the artificial light many of us encounter in the evenings of modern life.

Finally, the third component (in addition to melatonin and schedule shifting) is light exposure. It is crucial to ensure darkness during the sleep zone, either by light-blocking window shades or by wearing an eye mask to sleep. Then, upon awakening, that's when bright light exposure helps anchor the waking side of the rhythm. If light exposure occurs too early, before the planned wake time, then it can actually make things worse and further confuse the circadian rhythm. This is a problem for those severe night-owl types who try (or are told by someone) to "just get a lot of light" when they wake up. It is best, instead, to adjust the timing of morning light more gradually, with the schedule shifts we discussed above, since doing so is the most effective way to pull the brain's clock into the current time zone.

For morning-lark types, we use the same logic for the gradual movement of the sleep zone at a pace of thirty to sixty minutes every other day, but we reverse the timing of the light component of chronotherapy. The bright light is used in the evening, which helps push the clock back later in time. Melatonin is often not needed, as the evening light tends to be the main driver of the shifting for the morning lark types.

What about jet lag?

Jet lag may be the most common disturbance of the circadian system, and most of what has been written about jet lag has taken a purely circadian perspective. This focus makes sense, but we'll see in a moment that the homeostat is also part of the story. During westward travel, we're entering destination time zones that are earlier in clock time, so it feels as if we gain time before the clock strikes "bedtime" at our destination compared to our home time zone. After flying from New York to Los Angeles, 11:00 p.m. for our internal clock (aligned to the East Coast) would be only 8:00 p.m. on the West Coast clocks. Westward travel is generally easier to manage, as most people find it more natural to stay up a bit later to accommodate the destination time zone. That ability to stay up later is no accident, as most of us have a circadian rhythm that is slightly longer than twenty-four hours. Our inner clocks actually use cues like light exposure in the morning, as well as the timing of food and other exposures, to slightly "reset" the timing of our clocks each day, even when we are not traveling across time zones. If we did not do that (and some blind people cannot do this very well), then we would tumble forward through the twenty-four-hour clock continually, each day going to bed and waking up about ten minutes later because of the longer-than-twenty-four-hour inner rhythm.

Eastward travel across time zones, in contrast, tends to be harder for most people to adjust to. Again, because most of us have an inner rhythm slightly longer than twenty-four hours, it is less natural to go to bed earlier than usual. After flying from Los Angeles to New York, 11:00 p.m. at the destination is only 8:00 p.m. for our internal clock, which is still aligned to the West Coast, so we might not feel tired enough to hit the sack. We get a double whammy on the wake-up side as well: after having a hard time falling asleep earlier than usual, we also have to get up earlier than usual (for example, 7:00 a.m. in New York is 4:00 a.m. on the West Coast). The opposite morning issue happens for westward travel, which is another reason westward travel is easier to tolerate for most people (for example, 7:00 a.m. in Los Angeles is 10:00 a.m. on the East Coast).

Regardless of the direction of travel, the larger the time-zone change, the harder it is to adjust. Techniques to reduce jet lag usually involve adjusting the circadian system, but general tips such as maintaining hydration and avoiding alcohol are equally important. If schedules permit and a person is highly motivated, a gradual adjustment of sleep and wake times in the days leading up to travel across time zones can provide a running start to align with the destination zone. Websites such as www.jetlagrooster. com are freely available for customizing a travel plan to include sleep timing, light exposure, and the potential use (and timing) of melatonin supplements.

We started this chapter by talking about the two inner clocks that drive sleep-wake patterns. What about that second clock, the homeostat: Does it play a role? Of course! It could be just as important as the circadian system, especially if the flight lands in the evening at the destination time zone. For example, let's say a flight from the East Coast lands in California at 8:00 p.m. For someone who wishes to go to bed in the destination hotel at 10:00 p.m., this goal time would correspond to 1:00 a.m. in her home time zone, so it should theoretically be easy for her to fall asleep at that time—in fact, it could be hard to stay awake in the taxi to the hotel. But let's say this person falls asleep just after watching a movie early in the flight, and she slept for three hours straight, waking only with the jarring of the plane's wheels touching down. We wouldn't want to celebrate the magic of extra sleep so fast—that long nap might confuse the homeostat. In other words, when ten o'clock rolls around and she tucks into bed, the two clocks that are normally aligned at her bedtime are now in conflict: the circadian system is saying "It's late! Go to sleep!" while the homeostat is saying, "Hang on there—we just slept recently, so we're not tired at the moment." So for late-arriving flights at the destination, limiting sleep or getting it early in the flight may be a better plan. But keeping awake via caffeine on such flights may not be a great idea either, because it could last too long and, just like a long nap, also interfere with your sleep at your destination. For early-morning flights, catching some sleep on the flight can be helpful at your destination, where the homeostat will be on your side, with alertness at a peak to start the day.

One final word about context: this section about the homeostat assumes there hasn't been sleep deprivation leading up to the flight, and the flight was the only time he had to catch up—a competing need that might overtake any risk that this extra sleep might make it harder to get aligned at his destination. Jet lag stories can be isolated, like on vacation trips, or more frequent for those who travel for business or who work rotating shifts. With each person being differently sensitive to jet lag, light, caffeine, and naps, and having different obligations and flexibility for adjustments, managing the timing of sleep is a great example of balancing competing issues.

CHAPTER 16
My legs are restless

What causes restless legs syndrome?

Patients with restless legs syndrome, or RLS for short, report an uncomfortable sensation, usually in the legs, that is typically worse at night and that comes with an urge to move the legs, which provides some relief. RLS can interfere with falling asleep at the beginning of the night; it can also make falling back to sleep more difficult for those who awaken in the middle of the night. Depending on how severe it is, RLS can also cause sleepiness or impaired cognitive function during the day as a result of interfering with sleep. The symptoms can even occur during the day if people find themselves in situations in which their movement is restricted, such as during long car rides or during plane trips. Doctors make the diagnosis of RLS entirely based on the subjective symptoms (no sleep testing is required, but we'll talk about some exceptions later in the chapter). Now, that doesn't mean that making the diagnosis is easy. Many patients struggle with RLS symptoms for long periods of time, even years, because they may not know how to describe it, or they may not think of it as a medical problem or raise any concerns with their physician.

Exploring some of the causes is key to evaluating a patient with symptoms of RLS. Identifying one or more potentially reversible causes can go a long way toward improving symptoms. Of course, some of the risk factors are not modifiable, such as having a family history of RLS. Some situations that cause RLS are temporary, such as pregnancy, while others may be more permanent, such as certain forms of kidney disease. The most common cause that we can usually treat quite easily turns out to be a deficiency of iron. This can be investigated with a blood test called ferritin, which can be done at any doctor's office. The important detail here is that ferritin (and other iron related tests) are mainly done to look for anemia (low red blood cell counts), so the normal levels of ferritin are defined to diagnose anemia. In patients with RLS, it turns out that higher ferritin levels (compared to the levels required for making red blood cells) can be quite helpful for reducing RLS symptoms. In other words, we're looking for a relative kind of iron deficiency that is not necessarily enough to cause anemia. If the ferritin level isn't high enough, then taking iron pills (with some Vitamin C to help with absorption) can be a simple but effective treatment for RLS.

If the iron is not effective, or if the ferritin level was already high enough, then we can consider prescription options. But before we talk about medications, we need to make sure that other behavior modifications have been addressed. Just as we want to make sure sleep-hygiene tips[a] have been addressed before moving into more advanced treatments for patients with chronic insomnia, we want to make sure the low-hanging-fruit options have been considered for RLS patients before moving on to prescription treatments. For example, RLS can be worsened by alcohol, caffeine, and nicotine. Insufficient sleep for any reason can worsen RLS, so we want to make sure that sleep timing is regular and of adequate quantity and quality. Mild exercise or stretching or massage before bed can relieve or reduce symptoms. Certain medications can worsen RLS, such as antihistamines like diphenhydramine (which is an ingredient in several over-the-counter sleep aids), as well as antidepressants. Changing or stopping these medications, especially antidepressants, may or may not be feasible for a patient, so as usual we need to keep the patient's context in mind: balancing the severity of RLS symptoms against the flexibility to modify potentially contributing factors.

Patients and primary-care doctors differ in the stages at which they choose to obtain consultation with a sleep specialist for managing RLS. The next stage of medications, which are called dopamine agents, can be prescribed by primary-care doctors who are comfortable managing RLS. Other prescriptions involve additional risk-benefit discussions, and patients who move beyond dopamine agents may be more likely to have these discussions via consultation with a sleep clinic. There is even an FDA-approved device, called Relaxis, which uses vibration to alleviate the symptoms of RLS.

Do we need a sleep study to diagnose RLS?

To diagnose RLS, we only need to talk with the patient. This situation is similar to insomnia (which is based on symptoms, not testing), but unlike, say, sleep apnea,

---

a See chapter 6 for more on sleep hygiene.

where we must perform objective testing to make the diagnosis. When it comes to RLS, the patient's story is the whole story. There is no requirement to quantify the restlessness with sensors or measurements. But there is a closely related disorder called periodic limb movements of sleep, or PLMS for short. For that disorder, we do need to measure the leg movements objectively. Currently, testing for PLMS is only accomplished through laboratory polysomnography. The at-home testing kits that are becoming more popular are only used for detecting obstructive sleep apnea. They do not include the sensors required to measure leg movements. Several research groups have tried to measure PLMS using the same kind of motion sensors used in fitness trackers (called actigraphy), but they are placed on the ankles instead of the wrist.[100] Unfortunately the results were not impressive, so this technology has not yet enjoyed application in sleep clinics.

We might also consider polysomnography testing for a case of RLS that was either unusual or did not respond to treatments. The testing usually shows PLMS during sleep, which is known to occur in more than 85 percent of patients with RLS. That finding doesn't necessarily change the treatment options for RLS. What can change the treatment plan is if the patient turns out to also have sleep apnea, which can reduce sleep quality and indirectly worsen RLS symptoms.

I'll admit that PLMS is a tricky topic to deal with in clinical practice. Unless you have RLS symptoms, we don't have good clues or tools to predict who is at risk for elevated PLMS. That wouldn't be a big deal if PLMS only occurred in RLS patients (we can diagnose them just by their symptoms). But it turns out that the large majority of people with PLMS do not actually have RLS symptoms at all. They may have other symptoms of non-refreshing sleep (like sleepiness, or insomnia), but nothing necessarily that would point to a leg-twitching problem as a cause. Indirect information can sometimes provide a hint, such as when people notice changes in the covers or their body position when they wake up, but this is not so reliable because the movements can be quite subtle. Sometimes a bed partner notices the leg movements, if the movements are prominent enough—and if the bed partner is awake enough to make the observation.

In most cases, PLMS is discovered in a polysomnogram that was ordered to evaluate some other sleep complaint, such as sleepiness. While sometimes called an "incidental" finding, if that finding is the only abnormality observed on the test, and we have no better explanations for the patient's symptoms, then we might conclude that the PLMS are indeed the culprit disturbing sleep.

How aggressive we should be with trying to calm these twitches is currently a topic of debate. PLMS have not been studied nearly as well as other sleep problems such as sleep apnea. But some research suggests that PLMS are correlated with heart attack and stroke risks.[44] From research studies that measure the cardiovascular system more closely than is done in a typical polysomnogram, we can see that the leg twitches come with bursts of heart rate and blood pressure—the same fight-or-flight adrenaline kind of response we see with the breathing obstructions of sleep apnea. PLMS can prevent the normal overnight dip in blood pressure that happens as our bodies rest while sleeping. Although these studies raise important concerns, we still do not know for sure if PLMS cause health problems directly. In other words, we are at the correlation stage of evidence, but not yet at the causation stage. That's an important consideration, because if we could figure out whether PLMS actually cause these health problems, then we could consider treating PLMS for the sole purpose of reducing future health risks such as heart attack or stroke. Until then, decision making in the sleep clinic is driven mainly by the patient's symptoms. In that sense, the situation reminds us of how we used to think about sleep apnea in the past—that it was only worth treating if it were causing symptoms.[b]

If the data is so uncertain, how do we advise patients with PLMS?

Even though we don't yet know if treating the PLMS with iron pills or medications will reduce the risk of stroke and heart attack, we can still try to help each patient answer two fundamental questions: how worried should I be, and what are my options if I am worried enough to act. Let's assume that the patient has no sleep-related symptoms or RLS symptoms, so the only consideration is whether the PLMS pertains to heart attack and stroke risk. A patient who wanted to be very aggressive with therapy and was not risk averse when it comes to medications, might rationally choose to treat the PLMS (based on the available risk evidence we mentioned above), even if it is not standard clinical practice. Another patient, who might have less appetite for risk, might reasonably conclude that, in the absence of clear research evidence proving that treatment would be helpful, she should leave well enough alone.

Let's next think about a patient who feels that his sleep is non-refreshing and describes either insomnia or daytime sleepiness. Let's say we can't find an obvious cause during the clinical evaluation before testing is done, and the only finding on his polysomnogram testing is elevated PLMS. In this case, we might consider the PLMS

---

b See chapter 8 for more on the topic of sleep apnea and sleepiness.

as the potential cause of the symptoms, and we might thus decide it warrants treatment. Put another way, we have a direct and personalized hypothesis that, in this individual patient, the elevated PLMS are *causing* the sleep symptoms. Why am I hedging here that this is just a hypothesis? When we study large groups of people to learn more about PLMS, I admit that we don't see reliable clues to sort out whether, in general, PLMS are more likely to cause insomnia or sleepiness (or no symptoms at all). But there is enough reason to still try to connect the dots for an individual patient, through their own particular context, to come to decisions about whether or not to treat. This is a very practical approach: if we treat the PLMS, and the person feels better, then we may safely conclude that the legs were causing the symptoms. But what if treatment doesn't help the symptoms?

How can we tell if PLMS treatment is working?

With RLS, we can easily tell if the treatment is working: we simply ask people about their symptoms. For PLMS treatment, we also ask about symptoms, but if the symptoms are not getting better, we have to dig a bit deeper. Unless we conduct measurements, we wouldn't be able to tell whether or not the treatment was reducing the leg movements. If not, then the lack of *symptom* benefit could be because that medication was not working to reduce the leg movements for that patient. But if the leg movements were in fact reduced, but the patient still didn't feel any better about her sleep, then this might suggest that the leg movements were unrelated to the sleep symptoms. In other words, the leg movements were truly incidental findings on the polysomnogram. Technically speaking, even if the patient feels better with treatment, we would ideally still like to know whether the PLMS were actually reduced by the treatment. Feeling better with treatment is consistent with the hypothesis, but we can't rule out a placebo effect without measuring sleep objectively. Now, to be fair, the patient might not necessarily care if her improvement were thanks to placebo effect or not. But the statistical nerd in me wants to know: What portion of the symptom improvement was due to placebo and what portion was due to an actual treatment effect on reducing PLMS? In clinical practice, it is becoming harder and harder to obtain approval for in-lab polysomnography these days because of insurance restrictions that favor at-home kits (for detecting sleep apnea), so it's unlikely that we'd be performing repeated in-lab tests to guide treatment adjustments for PLMS. At least until we have home monitoring for these leg twitches, we'll depend on the patient's symptoms to assess therapy goals.

CHAPTER 17

Sleep perception—when the measurements don't match our experience

The dilemma of subjective versus objective sleep

The way sleep feels subjectively can be quite different from what the measurements of objective sleep testing say. This seems surprising because we expect a strong correlation between the two. Despite our gut sense telling us otherwise, many objective aspects of sleep turn out to be, at least in some people, disconnected from subjective sleep symptoms. Disconnection can mean an objective sleep problem is not causing symptoms, or can mean that subjective sleep symptoms are not showing up on objective sleep testing.

We shouldn't feel skeptical of the idea of disconnection of symptoms and physiology, between how something feels and what can be measured with testing. Some of the most common health problems cause no symptoms while they are gradually progressing until they finally "declare" themselves and cause an event. It's not hard to find examples of medical problems that do not always cause symptoms, or they may cause symptoms differently in different people. Even seemingly dramatic events such as heart attacks or strokes can cause a variety of symptoms, including being totally silent with no symptoms at all. Another common example is high blood pressure, which can develop silently and if untreated can eventually lead to a heart attack or a stroke. In modern medicine, aggressive screening for such problems makes sure we catch them in time rather than waiting for symptoms to arise. The very idea of screening recognizes that problems can exist before we feel anything at all.

These kinds of observations remind us that sleep is hardly unique among health topics for having the potential for the experience being different from the objective measurements. And just like finding out from an objective medical test that one has had a heart attack at some point in the past despite not having had any symptoms, it's not a question of the symptoms being right or wrong or a criticism of someone's ability to know her own body. Well, OK, sometimes it might be a question of right or wrong: How common is it to observe a family member doze off and start snoring and then deny he was snoring (or that he was sleeping), at least in the era before it was easy to record the evidence of snoring?

Even if we acknowledge certain aspects of health that can have a symptom-disconnect, it sure does seems as if sleep should *not* be like those other health problems. We can all decide how much weight to give the two key ingredients of subjective experience and objective measurements as we prepare to make decisions. If the experience and the data do not seem to align or agree, we can think about which one we should prioritize to help decision-making. The only "wrong" decision is if we ignore the fact that there are two key ingredients to consider!

On the other end of the subjective-objective spectrum, some medical disorders are actually defined entirely based on symptoms, and no objective tests are to be had in these cases; pain is an example. In such cases, a doctor may perform testing of some kind—not to prove or disprove the symptoms, but rather to look for potential causes that could be treated, such as whether a patient's back pain is from arthritis or from something more serious or urgent. Sleep problems feel closer to that kind of a problem than, say, to high blood pressure. How then should we think about sleep problems, somewhere between the two extremes of health problems defined entirely by symptoms versus health problems defined entirely by objective testing? What makes sleep challenging from a health perspective is not only that different sleep disorders involve different combinations of subjective and objective problems, but also that the combination can be quite different from person to person.

When it comes to sleep, it seems easy to feel defensive when we're presented with the idea that objective testing might be helpful, especially if the suspected problems are at odds with how sleep feels to us. Sleep is highly personal. Until I experienced the disconnect of feeling awake when the sleep sensors showed that I was clearly asleep,[a] I never would have believed that my impression of sleep could be so different from the measurements. The dilemma is that when a person's subjective and objective aspects of sleep are not aligned, it requires personal context to work through how much weight to give each one.

---

a See chapter 1 for some of my sleep story.

The two most common examples of subjective-objective mismatch in my sleep clinic

When patients come to my clinic with sleep concerns, and their experience matches up with the diagnostic testing, then decision-making is most straightforward. But any mismatches or disconnects can be barriers to decision-making. In the area of sleep apnea, the most common mismatch is when a person has little or no symptoms to suggest any breathing problems during sleep.[b] In other words, the mismatch is that she perceives her sleep to be of better quality than we observe with objective diagnostic measurements. In the area of insomnia, the most common mismatch is when a person perceives less sleep (or more time awake) during the night than we observe with objective diagnostic measurements. In other words, the mismatch is that he perceives his sleep to be worse than the measurements suggest. Two additional twists arise when it comes to chronic insomnia: we don't typically have objective measurements,[c] and when we do, sometimes we identify unexpected problems, such as sleep apnea.

To diagnose insomnia, I don't need a test to determine whether you have that symptom. But I would need a test to determine any potential degree of mismatch between objective measurements and your perception of time asleep and time awake. Again, it's not a matter of whether a person with insomnia is right or wrong when estimating sleep duration, any more than saying a feeling of hunger is right or wrong relative to a measure of actual caloric need. Insomnia is obviously a very real experience, just like hunger, or pain, or anxiety. Like these other experiences, which differ greatly between people, so the perception of sleep is a strikingly individual experience. What's important are the practical risk implications for insomnia patients who are sleeping more than they feel they are (as we discussed in chapter 13).

One form of mismatch or misperception occurs even in healthy adults with no sleep complaints: these folks tend to *overestimate* their sleep duration and continuity compared to what objective measurements tell us. They are not aware of the dozens of brief awakenings that always percolate throughout even a normal night of sleep. It is commonly, but mistakenly, thought that healthy sleep occurs in a solid, uninterrupted block (as we discussed in chapter 13). This mistaken thought could create a false sense of reassurance for a person who feels they sleep solidly but may have poor sleep quality (from, say, sleep apnea), or could create extra worry in the many people who awaken during the night and perceive those awakenings as definitively being unhealthy.

---

b See chapter 8 for more on disconnects between sleepiness and sleep apnea.

c See chapter 18 for more on diagnostic testing for patients with chronic insomnia.

I have to admit that I was amazed when I first learned about the disconnects between subjective and objective sleep, especially for chronic insomnia patients, where the diagnosis and management are based on self-reported sleep information. The differences between subjective perception and objective measurements of sleep duration were sometimes so striking and unexpected that I wondered if maybe we just weren't asking our questions about sleep symptoms in the best way. It turns out that how we ask about sleep does affect the answers people give,[26,27] but we still can't explain the fundamental question of how someone can feel wide awake while EEG sensors show typical brain wave patterns of normal sleep. We even thought that maybe we were placing the scoring labels incorrectly on the sleep-study data, or that the very definitions of sleep were incorrect—but this too, was a blind alley.[101] Some new research data suggests that different parts of the brain can be asleep versus awake at any moment in time—something that has been termed "local sleep."[102] Just as periods of brief sleep or drowsiness can intrude into our waking life, so can brief periods of wakefulness intrude into our sleep. We can hope that more advanced analyses such as machine learning (a component of what is now under the umbrella term, artificial intelligence) could help us make sense of the brain waves found on sleep EEGs to understand why some people "look" asleep to our sensors but feel awake.

Are there any risks to making decisions based solely on the perception of sleep?

If we consider our own experience and perception to be the gold standard when it comes to sleep, then how would that affect the risk-benefit balance when we make decisions about sleep health? For sleep apnea, we know that many people don't have typical symptoms, and so the condition can go undiagnosed and thus untreated.[d] For chronic insomnia, the situation is more interesting, because in clinical practice, the perception is accepted as the gold standard, and objective testing is not routinely sought. To be provocative, let's consider a person who strongly feels that he never sleeps, but when measurements are taken in a sleep lab, we find that not only is he sleeping most of the time he's in bed, but he also has a severe case of sleep apnea. Would we justify *not* offering treatment for sleep apnea because of the person's perception that he wasn't asleep, and thus he couldn't have sleep apnea? What if such a person never had a sleep test, but instead tried a sedative sleeping pill for the insomnia

---

d See chapter 8 for more on sleep apnea and sleepiness.

symptoms, and felt better about their insomnia symptoms, but was now masking or even worsening his sleep apnea? It seems like we'd want to avoid such a situation, not celebrate it as a treatment success. The point is that, given how much research has demonstrated disconnects between how sleep feels and what diagnostic measurements can show, we need to at least ask ourselves how much confidence we're willing to place in our own experience, and what potential risks could we encounter?

CHAPTER 18

Sleep testing—who, what, when, where, why, and how

Diagnostic polysomnography (PSG)

The standard in-laboratory testing night involves applying numerous sensors and wires to measure different aspects of sleep physiology. These include measuring brainwaves with scalp sensors (electroencephalogram, or EEG), muscle activity with sensors on the chin and legs (electromyogram, or EMG), eye movements with sensors near the eyes (electrooculogram, or EOG), and breathing patterns with a combination of belts around the chest and abdomen, oxygen sensing at the fingertip, and an airflow sensor placed just under the nose. In addition, the setup includes an electrocardiogram (ECG) sensor on the chest, a snoring sensor on the neck, and audio-video recording.

After the technologist applies the sensors, the lights are turned off, and the recording begins. Many patients are understandably concerned about their ability to sleep normally in such an unusual environment. The good news is that most people end up sleeping more than they think they will. After looking at thousands of nights of PSG recordings from our sleep testing center,[103] we found that the average amount of sleep is over six hours, from an average of 7.5 hours spent in bed for the test—not bad! Even for those who sleep much less than they usually would at home, in the vast majority of cases, the recording contains enough information to assess the most common sleep problems that bring patients to the lab for testing.

After the recording is completed, a sleep technologist reviews the entire night of data, in thirty-second segments or "epochs," and places scoring annotations into the record. The EEG, EOG, and chin EMG are used to assign sleep-wake stages to each epoch, according to a set of visual scoring rules. The current staging rules distinguish five stages: wake, rapid eye movement (REM) sleep, and three sub-stages of non-REM sleep (N1–3). Adults spend most of their sleep time in stage N2, followed by REM and N3 (also called deep or slow-wave sleep), both of which are about 20 percent of the night, and about 5 percent spent in stage N1. We'll come back to the stages at the end of this chapter.

The scoring technologist will also place annotations on the leg-muscle recordings to indicate twitching events. Because these twitches tend to occur with a certain rhythm, we've come to call them periodic limb movements of sleep (PLMS), which are summarized in an index of how many occur per hour of sleep (the periodic limb movement index, or PLMI). Most patients with restless legs symptoms during wakefulness also have PLMS after they fall asleep. Many more people, however, have PLMS activity that they don't even realize.[a]

The most common reason to test a person's sleep using overnight laboratory PSG is to make the diagnosis of sleep apnea, the most common form being obstructive sleep apnea. The scoring technologist places annotations on the breathing signals according to different types of breathing interruptions. The number that summarizes sleep apnea severity is called the apnea-hypopnea index, or AHI for short. This is the number of breathing interruptions per hour of sleep, and it provides an estimate of sleep apnea severity: fewer than five events per hour is normal, five to fifteen events per hour means mild sleep apnea, fifteen to thirty events per hour means moderate sleep apnea, and more than thirty events per hour is considered severe sleep apnea. Although different scoring conventions exist for the different types of interruptions, this summary index is the most commonly used metric of disease severity. The interruptions often (but not always) show a drop of oxygen of some degree, and most guidelines using an oxygen criteria suggest either 3 percent or 4 percent oxygen reductions.

In the early years of sleep-lab testing, patients who were found to have sleep apnea on their first PSG night would then return for a second night some days or weeks later to have a second night of PSG, this time while wearing a mask to deliver continuous positive airway pressure (CPAP) as treatment. This kind of PSG is called a CPAP titration, during which the patient tries different masks and pressures to determine the best treatment settings for their particular case of sleep apnea. In more recent years, most clinical testing centers have protocols to allow a trial both diagnosis and

a See chapter 16 for more on PLMS.

treatment settings to occur on a single PSG night. The decision to try CPAP in the second half of that night is based on whether the patient has had enough sleep apnea events in the first half (usually at least a moderate level is required). This is called a split-night study: the first part is the diagnosis or baseline portion, and the rest is the CPAP-treatment portion.

Testing for sleep apnea is by far the most common reason for PSG testing, and so it is not surprising that objective evidence of sleep apnea is the most common finding. Elevated PLMS is perhaps the next most common finding, occurring in 10-20% of people who undergo PSG testing. Beyond providing these common findings, using the wide variety of sensors we mentioned earlier in this chapter allows physicians to detect other problems such as teeth grinding (bruxism), heart-rhythm problems on the ECG sensor, abnormal behaviors in sleep (parasomnia), and in rare cases abnormal brain activity such as seizures.

Pros and cons of in-lab PSG

The comprehensive recording of in-lab PSG has the advantage of providing a very detailed and multisystem picture of a person's sleep. The level of detail is so high, in fact, that the field is still learning new ways to analyze the patterns. But even the traditional analysis methods provide important details that can help in making treatment decisions. Important examples include how much the sleep apnea changes according to sleep stage and body position, both of which can predict the response to different treatments, whether CPAP or an alternative treatment.[b] By analyzing all of the various aspects of sleep physiology, we are more likely to gain useful information that guides both making diagnoses and choosing treatment options, as well as ensuring that any unexpected or rare problems are ruled out.

The main downsides of in-lab PSG are related to the very same sensor system that gives us diagnostic advantages: the whole ordeal is expensive and inconvenient. Because the night spent in the sleep lab may not reflect a typical night at home, one concern is that the results may not be representative. In the sleep clinic, where sleep apnea is a common concern, it's important to consider night to night variability in the degree of breathing problem during sleep. Body position and alcohol are perhaps the two most common reasons that sleep can be different night by night. Since alcohol

---

b See chapter 11 for more on CPAP alternatives.

tends to disturb sleep and can increase sleep apnea interruptions, a night in the lab (without alcohol) might underestimate the level of the sleep problem (including sleep apnea) compared to a night at home when someone has consumed alcohol before going to bed. In the lab, patients are often asked to sleep at least part of the time on their back, which might not be their preference when sleeping at home. Since sleep apnea tends to be worse when sleeping on one's back, the measurements might seem worse in the lab compared to at home.[c]

Split night PSGs have their own set of pros and cons. The main advantage is that we get both the diagnosis and the treatment settings in a single night instead of two nights, thus saving time and cost. But one disadvantage is that the accuracy of the diagnosis, and the success of the pressure titration, may not be ideal because each is based on reduced amounts of time compared to dividing the process into two nights. As one example of how the information is limited, in about half of split-night PSGs in our center, REM sleep is not seen in the early part of the night used for diagnosis. Because sleep apnea is often worse during REM sleep, this means that we could be underestimating the severity of sleep apnea in these split-night PSGs that don't observe REM sleep in the first part. As another example, during the second part of a split-night PSG, the technologist may not have enough time to test the different pressure settings required to optimally correct the sleep apnea interruptions.

Home sleep apnea testing (HSAT) kits

These devices have only three or four sensors, compared to the larger set of sixteen to twenty sensors used during in-lab PSGs. Most of these kits have a belt that goes around the chest, which is connected to a sensor for oxygen and heart rate on the fingertip, as well as a sensor of airflow under the nose to measure breathing. In the last decade (since 2007 or so), HSAT device availability has grown substantially. The first official guidelines statement from the American Academy of Sleep Medicine on their use was published in 2007,[104] and in 2017 the academy released its updated guidelines.[58] HSAT kits are intended to be used in patients suspected of having the obstructive kind of sleep apnea, which is the most common kind. These devices usually have automated scoring software of some kind, which a sleep technologist reviews before a physician interprets the results.

---

c See chapter 11 for more on sleep apnea and body position.

Pros and cons of HSAT

The advantages of HSAT devices include their convenience and their low testing costs compared to in-lab PSGs. Although HSAT testing occurs in the comfort of one's home, technical problems are more likely to affect the testing without a "live" technologist monitoring the situation (such problems end up affecting about 10–15 percent of patients) . The main disadvantages relate to the same issue that makes these devices low-cost and convenient options: the limited number of sensors that are used. This trade-off means that leg movements are not measured, and in most of these kits, the brainwaves are not measured (no EEG sensors are used) and thus sleep stages are not monitored. Only some of these devices include body-position sensors,[105] which we mentioned a moment ago as important for characterizing sleep apnea. Taken together, these limitations cause HSAT devices to underestimate the severity of sleep apnea, especially in patients who have insomnia in addition to their sleep apnea.[63]

The repeated theme in this book is the importance of context, and the issue of in lab PSG versus at-home HSAT monitoring is another prime example of that.[d] For straightforward cases, where the suspicion is high that a person has significant obstructive sleep apnea, and the plan is to try CPAP therapy, then HSAT testing can be a fast and simple path to follow. But if someone is considering alternatives to CPAP (as in chapter 11), then the details of the sleep apnea diagnosis (also known as the sleep apnea phenotype[106,107]) can play a bigger role, and the limitations of HSAT kits become more problematic. The details like severity and position-dependence may help patients decide how worried they should be about their sleep apnea, including how motivated they should be about treatment, and if they choose treatment, to personalize the options. Of course, if we are considering sleep disorders other than sleep apnea, then the current HSAT devices simply don't provide the necessary information to do that. What we gain from HSAT kits in convenience and up-front cost savings we pay for in other ways: lower accuracy for diagnosing sleep apnea and its subtypes and failure altogether to detect problems other than sleep apnea.

Why isn't sleep testing performed for patients with insomnia?

It is not common for people with chronic insomnia to undergo objective measurements of sleep via PSG in a sleep lab. Why not? The reason is, in part, that the experience

---

d See chapter 9 for more on home testing for sleep apnea.

of insomnia is considered the gold standard for making the diagnosis, such that taking objective measurements is generally not deemed important unless another problem is suspected in addition to insomnia. The American Academy of Sleep Medicine guidelines state that PSG testing may be considered if the insomnia fails to respond to treatment or if the doctor has a reasonable suspicion of another sleep disorder that would require objective testing, such as sleep apnea or periodic limb movements of sleep. That seems straightforward, as long as we agree on what "reasonable suspicion" means. That's where things start to get interesting, so let's unpack this seemingly simple phrase as it relates to the common problem of sleep apnea.

First, we can rephrase the question of PSG testing in a more provocative way to frame the idea of reasonable suspicion: If you have chronic insomnia, then what chance of underlying sleep apnea would you be willing to ignore? If we don't perform testing, we might miss the diagnosis of sleep apnea, which gets back to the question of how to decide when suspicion of sleep apnea is reasonably high. Put another way, how low a chance is low enough to feel comfortable about putting the question to rest without testing? To answer this, we need to think about how we estimate a person's risk for sleep apnea. We usually think of important clues like obesity, snoring and gasping at night, and sleepiness during the day. But what if a person with chronic insomnia has none of those—are we reassured that the risk of sleep apnea is low enough to put it aside and forego testing? To answer this, we should consider some striking research on the overlap between sleep apnea and chronic insomnia.[45-48] It turns out that sleep apnea is common in people with chronic insomnia, even if they have none of the typical symptoms of sleep apnea. This is one set of research that really keeps me up at night, when I think of the millions of adults who take sleeping pills but have not ever had a PSG test.

That may be reason alone to think about the role of PSG testing. But let's dig a little deeper into this question of sleep apnea risk. Bear with a few percentages for a moment. If the adult population in America has a baseline risk of sleep apnea of, say, 10 percent, and we administer the best-validated screening tool called the STOP-Bang questionnaire (which is an acronym for the eight component questions), how should we interpret a positive screening test result? The positive screening means the chance of sleep apnea is higher than 10 percent (the baseline risk), but how much higher? It turns out that a positive screening only raises the risk from 10 percent to about 20 percent, because the screening is not perfect—far from it.[108] Despite this relatively small increase in risk, most health-care providers would say that a positive screening should cause us to be concerned enough to take a deeper look into sleep apnea, perhaps with an objective test. In other words, at a point somewhere between 10 percent and 20 percent, we've crossed a threshold of "enough" risk to take more action. Keeping this screening situation in mind, let's now revisit insomnia. If we believe that the data we mentioned earlier, showing increased sleep apnea risk in chronic insomnia patients, then the diagnosis of chronic insomnia itself suggests an even higher risk of sleep apnea than is the case from a positive sleep apnea screening test applied among the general adult population. In other words, we could build the argument that the presence of chronic insomnia itself is enough to give us reasonable suspicion of sleep apnea.

In-lab CPAP titration versus at-home automatic titration

We can also consider the trade-offs between in-lab and at-home options for treating sleep apnea with CPAP. In-lab titration has the advantage of offering detailed data collection and real-time technologist adjustments, which in combination will help the physician arrive at a confident plan for CPAP treatment settings. If the mask becomes difficult to tolerate during the night, then the technologist can make adjustments to the mask and headgear as well. But these advantages also make the night in the lab costly. Using an automatically adjusting CPAP machine, or auto-CPAP, can be a low-cost and convenient alternative to in-lab CPAP titration. The American Academy of Sleep Medicine published the initial clinical guidelines for these devices a decade ago (in 2008).[109] The at-home pathway to treatment begins with an auto-CPAP machine, and if this is not effective or tolerated, then the patient can consider an in-lab CPAP titration. As is the case with HSAT devices at the diagnosis phase of the process, auto-CPAP machines at the treatment phase of the process are intended for straightforward cases of obstructive sleep apnea. In other cases, such as central apnea, complex apnea, or other breathing problems, auto-CPAP may not be effective or appropriate.[e]

Daytime nap tests: multiple sleep latency and maintenance of wakefulness tests

The typical test for patients with excessive sleepiness, also called hypersomnia, is the multiple sleep latency test (MSLT). This test is performed mainly for patients who are suspected of having narcolepsy or sleepiness of unknown causes, which is also

---

e See chapters 10 and 11 for more on the different treatments for breathing in sleep.

known as idiopathic hypersomnia. The idea is straightforward: people are given five nap opportunities spread throughout the day every two hours, and if they have excessive sleepiness, then they'll fall asleep more quickly than is normal, on average, during these nap opportunities (we typically use a cut-off value of eight minutes to fall asleep). In cases of narcolepsy, we observe in addition to fast sleep onset that REM sleep occurs on the recordings during at least two of the naps. In contrast, patients with idiopathic hypersomnia do not typically have REM sleep during these naps, but they still fall sleep more quickly than normal.

Because certain disturbances of sleep, including insufficient sleep duration, can cause hypersomnia, it is routine to perform an in-lab PSG the night before the MSLT to (1) make sure the person does not have sleep apnea and (2) to ensure that he or she has gotten at least six hours of sleep prior to the day of nap testing. Another twist to the MSLT test is that the patient should not be on certain medications for two to four weeks leading up to the nap day, including stimulant drugs (such as amphetamine-class drugs, or the non-amphetamine drug modafinil) and antidepressant drugs (including older agents used as sleeping pills, such as trazodone). If a person stops his daily stimulant medication abruptly—say, the day of the nap study—then rebound sleepiness can occur and make the nap results appear even worse (faster sleep onset). The antidepressant medications can suppress REM sleep, and since the diagnosis of narcolepsy relies on observing REM sleep during some of the naps, these medications can affect the diagnosis of narcolepsy by the MSLT.

A related but less commonly used test is the maintenance of wakefulness test (MWT for short). Unlike the protocol for the MSLT, where patients are instructed to try to sleep and are lying down in a dark room, for the MWT protocol the patient is sitting up and is instructed to try to remain awake. We can conclude that, the longer she is able to maintain wakefulness, the less sleepy she is. The MWT is not performed for any particular diagnosis but rather to quantify a person's ability to stay awake, typically for individuals with concern for sleepiness behind the wheel or on the job. It is unclear, however, if this test mimics drowsiness risk in real-world settings such as during long drives or while working at a job for which dozing off could present serious risk.

Actigraphy

This technique has been used for decades to track sleep-wake patterns by sleep researchers.[110] Actigraphy also became popular in consumer sleep-monitoring devices since about 2005, and is still used today in this area.[38] The idea is that, for most people, when they are awake, they tend to move around, and while they are asleep, they tend not to move as much, so measuring motion with a wearable device can track these patterns. Because actigraphy devices do not directly measure whether the brain is asleep or awake, people working in the sleep field often refer to them as rest-activity monitors rather than sleep-wake monitors. For example, someone who's awake could be sitting or lying very still, and in this circumstance, the monitor might mistake the motionless awake time as sleep. Sometimes the reverse can occur: actigraphy could mistakenly indicate awake time in someone who's actually sleeping, as one study showed for someone sleeping on a bus.[111]

Sleep stages

The REM and non-REM sleep stages are front and center in most books about sleep. But they appear at the end here, and that's for a simple reason: despite the elegant (if not slow-paced) history of the discovery of the different sleep stages, in the real world of clinical practice, the stages during overnight PSG do not commonly translate into specific treatment recommendations. For those circumstances in which stages *do* play a role, it is usually not in the way in which stages seem to be discussed in the media. I'll be the first to admit that it's enticing to think about enhancing our cognitive function or fending off diseases of the brain by boosting REM sleep or deep sleep. Many thoughtful and accomplished researchers are working to move these ideas forward.[112-115] But the part of me that needs to help patients make practical and real-world decisions for their health is very preoccupied by sleep apnea, insomnia, and other treatable sleep disorders. That's why most of this book is about addressing common sleep health questions and disorders, figuring out how worried you should be, and determining where you should put your energy if you're going to make changes to improve your sleep situation.

Let's think through how these different perspectives sometimes play out in the sleep clinic. Even if I thought it were medically proven that increasing REM sleep or boosting deep non-REM sleep would improve mental or physical health, we do not yet have reliable methods to do so directly. Some treatments may do this indirectly, however, by removing a problem that was interfering with normal sleep stages. A common example is that some patients with sleep apnea experience a rebound of REM sleep when they first sleep with a CPAP mask, as if the brain had been keeping track of missing out on normal REM cycling. This REM effect is not, however, consistent from patient to patient, and we don't treat sleep apnea to achieve this effect. Truth be told, I spend more time worrying about the disorders associated with REM sleep than its health benefits. The main example is that sleep apnea tends to be worse during REM sleep, so much so that researchers have tried to use medications to suppress REM sleep as a treatment for sleep apnea.[116] This approach turns out not work consistently, for reasons unrelated to any link between REM and cognition, though it is possible that future studies will predict which sleep apnea patients are likely to respond.[117] Less common disorders such as acting out dreams physically (known as REM behavior disorder) and narcolepsy involve abnormalities in REM sleep that cause troublesome symptoms, some of which we treat with REM-suppressing medications. Not that long ago, because nearly all antidepressant medications suppress REM, the psychiatric research literature was suggesting that REM sleep increased the risk for depression, and that the medications for depression worked because they suppressed REM sleep.[35] This gap between research and clinical practice extends beyond sleep stages. For example, during non-REM sleep, the EEG shows brief events called sleep spindles, which have been linked to cognitive function in research studies,[118,119] but spindles still do not enjoy any special status in clinical practice; they are neither scored by the technologists nor reported in a physician's interpretation of a PSG test.

A clinical session doesn't go by in which I'm not reminded of how the gaps between the research world and the real world can affect patient care and decision-making. If everyone really agrees that sleep stages are so crucial for memory, then how can we reconcile that with the fact that REM is suppressed by common medications taken by millions of adults without any obvious cognitive consequences?[120] One potential way to reconcile this is to speculate that research studies involve such carefully controlled conditions that the discovered effects simply aren't easy to recognize in more real-world settings.[37] I spend more time in the clinic trying to redirect conversations to practical treatment decisions than on discussing how much REM or deep non-NREM sleep happened to have occurred on the night someone spent in the sleep lab. Patients are often in disbelief that they've been taking medications that suppress REM sleep—including some sleeping pills—because they had heard from other sources that REM was so important for them. They may have been even more frustrated about sitting in front of a sleep neurologist who didn't seem concerned about their REM sleep amounts. When I interpret PSG results in my clinic, I find that the sleep stages may be the least interesting thing about the night. If I only look at the sleep stages of a PSG, then I cannot make even the slightest guess as to what diagnosis may be present, what symptoms may be present (for example, insomnia or excessive daytime sleepiness), or even whether the patient may think they were awake or asleep during the night.[f]

If we take a step back from questions about the importance of difference sleep stages, we must admit to ourselves (if we are honest) that we don't really know if our current scoring rules for assigning the different sleep stages are "correct" in a biomedical sense, or whether, instead, other features of sleep physiology might be more important to health, such as heartbeat patterns[121] or sleep-wake transitions.[122,123] The history of assigning sleep stages to overnight EEGs dates back to the 1930s for non-REM, whereas REM was first identified in 1953.[14] The first widely accepted scoring manual, which defined one kind of REM sleep and four sub-stages of non-REM sleep, was published in 1968.[124] That scoring approach remained in place until 2007, when the American Academy of Sleep Medicine decided to combine the third and fourth non-REM stages into a single "deep" stage, called N3.[125] These original and revised scoring decisions were based on expert consensus opinion of visual patterns observed during PSG, rather than a specific medical reason or health consequence guiding the assignment of staging rules.

As a sleep physician, I often remain quietly frustrated, as I'm sure my patients are, that the excitement about sleep stages in the research world do not earn a prominent place in clinical practice conversations. Maybe the problem is that I sometimes see patients who are too complicated: they have other problems that muddy the waters, and a story about their sleep stages and cognitive function really is buried in there somewhere and ready to be told. How much are we willing to dig for that story? If we peel away the complicating factors of medications, health problems, and sleep disorders, we're still left with two key hurdles related to variability. First, since just about every aspect of sleep that can be measured varies from person to person,[49] it stands to reason that any link between sleep stages and waking function will also vary from person to person. Second, just about every aspect of sleep that can be measured also varies from night to night within a single person. We could overcome both hurdles if we could measure sleep stages accurately over multiple nights, and people tracked or measured aspects of daily life they were interested in finding links with their own particular sleep patterns. With the explosion of consumer sleep-tracking devices,[g] the opportunity to measure sleep is theoretically possible, if their validation can be improved.[38]

---

f See chapter 17 for more on sleep perception.

g See chapter 4 for more on consumer sleep trackers.

CHAPTER 19

Knowledge and discovery

Self-discovery

We don't need large research studies to tell us what we know from everyday life: people have different stories when it comes to every aspect of sleep, from different sensitivities to coffee and different abilities to nap, to different preferences for what time to sleep and for how long. Even within individual people, not every cup of coffee provides the same boost and not every nap is magically refreshing. Sleep quantity and quality can also vary from night to night, even in the most regimented of sleepers. When I worked on a textbook chapter to summarize the research literature's findings about using caffeine and naps as countermeasures against sleepiness,[51] I remember feeling overwhelmed at how variable things were, even in research studies that had been designed to remove (or control) as many variables as possible to make the experiments "clean" and thus easier to interpret. When we examine other common questions (such as how exercise or a natural supplement might help sleep), we face the same challenge: a striking amount of variability from person to person. Then, add to this variability the fact that people might perform different types of exercise at different times of day, and for different durations or intensities. Natural supplements may differ in potency and dosage. The literature reveals that variability is common,[49,126] including susceptibility to sleep deprivation,[127-129] vulnerability to sleepiness in sleep apnea,[60] altered perceptions of sleep,[72] sensitivity to the alerting effects of caffeine[52] and naps,[51,130] and sensitivity to the sedating effects of alcohol.[131] It is daunting for a researcher to consider the possibilities.

Variability not only complicates interpretation of the scientific literature (not to mention performing scientific research), but also makes it challenging for individuals to figure out their own patterns by trial and error. Keeping a sleep-wake diary is a natural step toward self-discovery, and the American Academy of Sleep Medicine guidelines suggest what factors to track in such a diary.[50,132,133] However, beyond using a qualitative review of diary entries, no accepted methods have been proposed for interpreting the diary patterns. If someone is very sensitive to something like coffee (in terms of it having a major impact on his sleep), he might have figured that out without keeping a detailed diary, or if he did keep a diary, he wouldn't need much in the way of special analysis to help find the pattern. But what about the more common reality: many behaviors and experiences during the day affect our sleep, and poor sleep is not the only thing that can sap our energy during the day. Teasing out patterns when many variables are in play can be tricky. Personal context and even recent sleep behaviors can matter quite a bit. Let's take an extreme example: someone who typically gets good energy from a regular cup of coffee. But then, one day, she pulls an all-nighter to work on a last-minute deadline. That same cup of coffee, consumed at the same time in the morning, now can't stop her from dozing, because it's fighting a different fight: a full night of sleep loss! In the daily ebb and flow of life, even without such extreme examples like all-nighters, sorting through possible patterns related to sleep quantity or quality can be, well, exhausting.

In the research world, when we want to test an idea—say, that yoga improves sleep quality—we'd typically design an experiment that would remove or control behaviors that could muddy the waters. We might ask research subjects to abstain from caffeine, alcohol, naps, or other forms of exercise besides yoga, and to keep a regular sleep-wake schedule of bedtime and morning alarms. The point of these (perhaps onerous) rules is to increase the chance of finding an effect of yoga on sleep, and is reasonable from a scientific perspective. But in the real world, not many of us live such controlled lives. We might even have routines that we are unable or unwilling to change. Think about someone who only takes naps on weekends (which in some people can make sleep worse) but also only has time to exercise on the weekends (which in some people can make sleep better). Now let's say she wants to try acupuncture to help improve her sleep, but she only has time to go to the acupuncturist on the weekends. You can see how this real-world setting is quite different from how we would want to design an experiment. In a research test of acupuncture effects, we would want to avoid competing with naps and exercise (which were, in her case, competing with each other already for possible effects on sleep).

Is there a way to use research-design principles in the real world? Let's say you have a lot going on in your life, and each day of the week is peppered with a different combination of caffeine, naps, alcohol, exercise, and stress. Say you wanted to see if the latest herbal sleep remedy could improve your sleep. How long would you have to try it? If it had a "gangbuster" benefit for you, then maybe you'd notice right away. But even prescription sleeping pills can't often boast such major sleep benefits. If the effect is less obvious, which is far more commonly the case, then it could get lost in the "noise" of all the other things going on that could be affecting your sleep from night to night. In that case, one solution would be to keep track of things for a long period of time to tease apart the "signal" (of the herbal) from the "noise" (of life). How long to track depends on how big of an improvement you're interested in finding and how variable your sleep-wake experience is from night to night. Large effects in a person with stable sleep patterns from night to night can be detected fairly quickly, maybe within a week. But the smaller the effect, and the larger the person's nightly variability is in general, the longer it will take to convincingly detect the effect at all. If the answer to "how long" seems to be an overly long time, then you might consider actively simplifying your daily experience to reduce the variability in behaviors we can control such as naps and caffeine and alcohol. In other words, you must make trade-offs between how many variables potentially affect your sleep on a given day, how much variability occurs from day to day within each behavior, how much improvement you desire to get from the herbal, and your willingness to keep track of things for extended periods of time. Only very large or obvious effects and correlations can be detected by tracking things for one to two weeks. If you are willing to search for more realistic effects (which tend to be less obvious), then tracking yourself for longer periods of time can take some serious commitment.[a]

Let's go back just for a moment to the idea of qualitatively looking over a diary for patterns. Let's say you enjoy coffee, but you've been struggling lately with insomnia symptoms and are well aware that caffeine could be playing a role, especially when you consume it later in the day. Now let's say you track yourself for a week or two, but you don't notice any clear patterns in how bad your sleep was after the days when you happened to have coffee after dinner. We might not want to conclude that the coffee had no effect just yet; we'd need to know something about the rest of the diary as well as how many other factors could have added noise to the patterns. It could still be that coffee is hurting your sleep but is only part of a bigger picture that made this effect

---

a To provide some guidance in pattern discovery, we made a free online tool: www.guidedselftesting.com. It's not a diagnostic test; it is a way to look for patterns in sleep-wake diaries and rank them by how large they are (statistically speaking), including estimated duration of tracking to find effects of different sizes.

hard to appreciate. It's easy to see how teasing these things apart can be a daunting task and why either tracking ourselves for longer periods of time, or actively trying to simplify competing factors from our lives, could be useful options for those who are motivated to discover patterns.

Making the leap from research world to real world

In the era of evidence-based medicine and precision medicine, patients are increasingly taking the reins with their own research into health topics. Whether through increased awareness and patient-advocacy groups or through increased access to online sources of information about the latest research, health information is now more available to the general public than ever before. From the patient's perspective, however, interpreting the latest research is not always straightforward. If physicians and researchers disagree about common and basic questions in sleep medicine (which they do), then this should serve as a reminder of how important it is for each of us as individuals to consider context when making sleep-health decisions. Personalizing health-care decisions is not just a buzzword—it is a necessity.

Two terms used in medical research describe the challenges of extrapolating findings from the research world and applying them to the real world. As we discussed in chapter 4, we use the term "external validity" to describe the extent to which findings in a specific population may be extended to another population. For example, if you perform a study of men, how confidently can you extend the study's findings to women? The answer would depend on information like how differently the disease manifests in men versus women and how differently men versus women respond to therapy. We use the term "ecological validity" to describe the extent to which the findings of a research study can be extrapolated to real-world environments. In other words, even if the target population in the real world is the same as that which was studied in the original experiments, would the findings still hold up without the structure and support of being enrolled in a research protocol? For example, an experiment that's performed in a sleep laboratory in which a new device is shown to be able to detect sleep apnea with a high level of accuracy may not perform as well when the device is tested in the home environment. This difference could have occurred because of challenges in proper application of the device or because some aspect of the home environment differed from that of the lab (and the device performance is vulnerable to that aspect), such as type of bedding, the presence of a bed partner, or room humidity.

One interesting example of how challenging it can be to extrapolate findings from the research world to the real world, and from groups to individuals, has to do with CPAP treatment and weight gain. If you want to scare people away from a treatment, tell them that it could cause weight gain. Oddly enough, it's true that some studies have reported weight gain in those who use CPAP treatment for sleep apnea. Although many theories have been proposed as to why this may be, researchers still don't fully understand whether a change in metabolism or a change in dietary patterns explains why weight changes with CPAP treatment of sleep apnea. Let's look at the details of one large study[134] that reported that those study participants who had been randomized to receive treatment with CPAP gained an average of 0.35 kilograms, or about twelve ounces, during the study. The error range on that average estimate of weight gain was more than five kilograms, or eleven pounds. The average weight gain was relatively small, while the margin of error was by comparison very large, which means that some people actually experienced substantial weight *loss*, while others gained much more than the average of twelve ounces. For someone who's concerned about the relation of CPAP use to weight gain, the average change in a group is arguably less important than answering the question: Am I more likely to be in the major weight-gain or the major weight-loss range of that bell curve? Thinking just about the *average* weight gain provides a very limited view of what can happen, yet we need to provide context to people to help them make very personal decisions.

Admittedly, we might not be able to answer that question, and predict the weight change for an individual. But we can rephrase the perspective and ask: If my sleep apnea is bad enough, and I'm able to adhere to CPAP therapy, then are the benefits of treatment to my quality of life and overall health sufficient, such that I'd actually accept some potential for weight gain? This is the question people have to ask themselves, and maybe being aware of the potential risk, they could think about steps to avoid weight gain happening. We see similar kinds of trade-offs in other health decisions: by analogy, many people report some weight gain after quitting cigarette smoking. We can frame the question of smoking with the same kind of personalized risk-benefit balance: How much weight gain would I accept, given the health benefits of quitting cigarette smoking? Each smoker would answer somewhat differently. Some people might be turned off from quitting smoking by the prospect of weight gain, which would be like and saying: "The idea of weight gain is so negative to me that I'm willing to accept the numerous known risks of continuing to smoke." Since many techniques can be used to maintain weight, it seems that standing behind such a statement would be challenging, no matter how frightening weight gain can seem, since the health consequences of smoking are themselves so frightening.

Trials and tribulations

For those patients with insomnia who are considering a sleeping pill, the discussion with their physician always includes the topic of side effects. It's worth taking a moment to ask: How do we doctors learn about the side effects of medications? It turns out to be less of a clear path than we'd hope. For the most part, we learn from the same kinds of studies that test for treatment benefits, which also keep track of adverse effects. Although in rare cases the goal of the study is to specifically test adverse effect rates, in most cases, the adverse effects are gathered while the researchers are conducting a study designed primarily to test the good effects of a medication. Here's where a bit of statistics will help understand why this tag-along approach is complicated. Adverse effects usually occur less frequently, on average, than good outcomes (thankfully!). When studies are designed with the good effects of medication in mind, they are most likely not large enough to quantify the adverse effects (which are less likely to be observed) as adequately as they quantify the good effects. In statistical parlance, this means that most studies tend to be "underpowered" to detect adverse events, especially the rare ones. Since the most severe adverse effects are typically rare (fortunately), this means that we're most vulnerable to mis-quantifying the most severe kinds of medication risks in typical research studies. One way to address this problem is through a process known as "post-marketing surveillance", basically watching for problems once a drug is FDA approved, because many more people are exposed to a drug once it's approved compared to during clinical trials performed to gain approval. This area of research has suggested multiple adverse risks of sleeping pill use, ranging from infections to cancer to dementia—even increased risk of mortality.[78] These risks are fortunately not common. Since we're unlikely to be able to conduct proper randomized trials for certain questions (such as the risk of rare but serious side-effects), it's even more important that patients and doctors have candid discussions of how to put treatment decisions in context for each individual.

Post-marketing surveillance has the benefit of involving a sufficiently large population to understand how common adverse events may be, but it still has one key weakness: it can't answer the crucial question of causality. To know for certain that a drug causes something (good or bad), we need to randomly assign research study volunteers to get either the treatment or the placebo. But it is much more difficult to randomize very large groups for the purpose of side effects, so post-marketing surveillance is the next best option despite the uncertainties that remain about causality.

If you feel like we're overthinking things and making them too complicated, you're not alone, but humor me for one more example. Let's take a common situation to illustrate the distinction between correlation and causation. Say you'd like to understand whether people with obstructive sleep apnea have fewer heart attacks if they use CPAP treatment compared to not using CPAP. Then say you round up one hundred people who use CPAP regularly, and then you find another hundred people who do not currently treat their sleep apnea. After five years, it turns out that fewer heart attacks happened in the "using CPAP" group. We'd like to conclude, since the untreated group had more heart attacks, that CPAP reduces heart attack risk. Not so fast! We've shown a correlation, but we haven't shown causation, because the treatment, CPAP, was not randomly assigned. In other words, the group using CPAP could be different from the untreated group in important ways, and those differences could account for the reduction in heart attacks, rather than the CPAP. Maybe the group using CPAP was more observant of other health-promoting behaviors such as exercise, weight loss, or compliance with medications. If so, we can't tell whether CPAP has a benefit of reducing heart attack risk or whether using CPAP is simply an indicator of healthy behaviors in general, and those other healthy behaviors (besides CPAP use) actually caused the reduced heart attack risk. In reality, it is probably a mixture of both. Although we can debate whether teasing this distinction apart is important or not from the patient perspective, we must concede that we have not established causality without performing a randomized trial that assigned treatment pathways (rather than people choosing treatment pathways themselves).

Sleep and health: turning a vicious cycle into a virtuous cycle

Sometimes health problems become overwhelming: How do we prioritize battles in what seems like a war with multiple fronts? A person might, after reflection, decide that "I want to focus on my diabetes first, and then I'll worry about my sleep." For someone who's grappling with a growing list of medications, including insulin injections, introducing a nightly routine of sleeping with a mask to treat sleep apnea might understandably seem like too much to worry about. But if the diabetes remains hard to control, one reason for this could be the very fact that the sleep apnea has gone untreated. If so, then a decision to first focus on the diabetes is an uphill battle at risk for failure. Even when an obvious-appearing relationship can be found, such as pain causing sleep disturbances ("A causes B"), feedback loops with sleep can create a vicious cycle: sleep disturbance worsens pain ("B causes A"). We might consider similar cycles for anxiety or depression, where sleep problems can be both cause and effect. All patients bring different perspectives to where they think they can put their energy to best use. One way to frame such decisions is to turn the vicious cycle into a positive cycle of better sleep and better health. That could simply mean simultaneously working on improving sleep and pain (or other health problem), instead of trying to decide which one is really causing the other. The cycle idea, of sleep and other health problems being both cause and effect for each other, is more commonly the case. And making headway on either front may benefit the other, and in this way the vicious cycle is flipped into a virtuous cycle[b].

---

b Our online tool, mentioned earlier in the chapter, helps identify these kinds of cycles in diary-tracking data (www.guidedselftesting.com)

CHAPTER 20

Epilogue

Although we look to science and research to explain what we don't understand, the scientific process is by nature uncertain. The self-correcting nature of scientific discovery is imperfect, and when self-correction does happen, it may happen slowly and may not enjoy the excited welcome typically earned by the novelty of being first. This reality introduces the potential for unintended consequence in the form of selective referencing of research findings that can best support a line of current reasoning. The optimistic interpretation is that experts see the forest for the trees well enough to prioritize what is important and can curate a summary of evidence that will lead to the prioritized conclusions. The pessimistic interpretation is that selective referencing can make an idea sound far more convincing than it should be, which has earned the derogatory term "cherry-picking." Most of the time, if cherry-picking occurs, it is to defend some important aspect of sleep to improve health. But I can build a case for REM sleep being bad for us by focusing on the benefits of REM-suppressing medications, or by highlighting that certain sleep disorders occur only in REM, examples of which include REM behavior disorder and some forms of sleep apnea. I can prove that, for some patients with sleep apnea, CPAP treatment actually makes their breathing worse. I can quote dozens of very large studies that have shown that getting too much sleep is actually worse than getting too little sleep in terms of health risks.

The point is that, by anchoring ourselves to the recurring theme of interpreting medical evidence in a personal context, we can at least insulate ourselves from the overconfidence of cherry-picked narratives. We can then reason through uncertainty when we have to make decisions for ourselves in the face of complicated sets of facts, or honest disagreement among experts, or the field of sleep medicine simply having incomplete information. The point is that, in sleep medicine, with so many points of uncertainty, it's safe to assume that you'll only find the "right" answer for you as an individual from placing the information in the personal context of your sleep story.

Hopefully you have not picked this chapter as the first one to read, in which case the last two paragraphs will probably have seemed too pessimistic. If you've read at least some of the other chapters before coming to this one, hopefully you've felt that the uncertainty in sleep medicine was balanced by practical ideas to help make real-world decisions about sleep health. Now, to balance out that philosophical epilogue, below I've given a brief list of further online resources about sleep health. There are many others of course, and most major hospitals have a sleep division web site with patient-focused information.

The American Academy of Sleep Medicine: The academy web site includes most current "practice guideline" articles for a variety of sleep disorders. (The target audience is medical professionals, but the content is open).

https://aasm.org/clinical-resources/practice-standards/practice-guidelines

The AASM also provides information for a general audience at: *www.sleepeducation.org.*

Several groups provide information on all aspects of sleep, targeted for a general audience.

The National Sleep Foundation: *https://sleepfoundation.org*
The American Sleep Association: *www.sleepassociation.org*

Other general health and medical sites include sleep disorder information such as *www.webMD.com* and *www.UpToDate.com* (which is a paid service for medical professionals, but has patient-centered options (*www.uptodate.com/home/uptodate-subscription-options-patients*). The National Institutes of Health (NIH) has extensive online resources, including a portal dedicated to research studies (*www.clinicaltrials.gov*).

Several sites are available that focus on specific sleep health topics:

Sleep Apnea
www.MyApnea.org (a large online community of patients and physicians)
www.sleepapnea.org (the Sleep Apnea Association)

Restless Legs Syndrome: *www.rls.org*

Hypersomnia: *www.hypersomniafoundation.org*

Narcolepsy: *www.narcolepsynetwork.org*, and *www.wakeupnarcolepsy.org*

Society for Behavioral Sleep Medicine: *www.behavioralsleep.org*

Many research publications are from journals with paywalls, so if you are not affiliated with an academic intuition with subscription access, you'll need to pay a fee to read beyond the abstract, unfortunately. Another option is to contact the author(s) and request a PDF reprint by email (most authors are exuberant to learn that anyone is interested in reading their work). Making journal articles open access is becoming more common—below are some examples of review articles that anyone can access online (typically through a portal called PubMedCentral, *www.ncbi.nlm.nih.gov/pmc/*). In the reference section at the end of this book, I've also highlighted which articles are open access, with a bolded web address, for those interested in digging deeper. Even though some articles (maybe most!) have more jargon specific to a research audience, the "Introduction" and "Discussion" sections typically contain more easily digestible content.

"(Mis)perception of sleep in insomnia: A puzzle and a resolution."
www.ncbi.nlm.nih.gov/pmc/articles/PMC3277880/
"Urgent Need to Improve PAP Management: The Devil Is in Two (Fixable) Details."
www.ncbi.nlm.nih.gov/pmc/articles/PMC5406947/

REFERENCES

1. McEvoy RD, Antic NA, Heeley E, et al. "CPAP for Prevention of Cardiovascular Events in Obstructive Sleep Apnea." *N Engl J Med* 2016;375:919-931.
    www.ncbi.nlm.nih.gov/pubmed/27571048

2. Memo. 2017. (Accessed March 10, 2017, at www.acgmecommon.org/announcement.)

3. Bilimoria KY, Chung JW, Hedges LV, et al. "National Cluster-Randomized Trial of Duty-Hour Flexibility in Surgical Training." *N Engl J Med* 2016;374:713-727.
    www.ncbi.nlm.nih.gov/pubmed/26836220

4. Watson NF, Martin JL, Wise MS, et al. "Delaying Middle School and High School Start Times Promotes Student Health and Performance: An American Academy of Sleep Medicine Position Statement." *J Clin Sleep Med* 2017;13:623-625.
    www.ncbi.nlm.nih.gov/pmc/articles/PMC5359340/

5. Marx R, Tanner-Smith EE, Davison CM, et al. "Later school start times for supporting the education, health, and well-being of high school students." *Cochrane Database Syst Rev* 2017;7:CD009467.

6. Watson NF. "Sleep duration: a consensus conference." *J Clin Sleep Med* 2015;11:7-8.
    www.ncbi.nlm.nih.gov/pmc/articles/PMC4262955/

7. Youngstedt SD, Goff EE, Reynolds AM, et al. "Has adult sleep duration declined over the last 50+ years?" *Sleep Med Rev* 2016;28:69-85.
    www.ncbi.nlm.nih.gov/pubmed/26478985

8. Editor. "Sleeplessness." *British Medical Journal* 1894;2:719.

9. Cowie MR, Woehrle H, Wegschelder K, et al. "Adaptive Servo-Ventilation for Central Sleep Apnea in Systolic Heart Failure." *N Engl J Med* 2015;373:1095-1105.
    www.ncbi.nlm.nih.gov/pubmed/26323938

10. Ohayon M, Wickwire EM, Hirshkowitz M, et al. "National Sleep Foundation's sleep quality recommendations: first report." *Sleep Health* 2017;3:6-19.
    www.sciencedirect.com/science/article/pii/S2352721816301309?via%3 Dihub

11. Pelayo R. "Commentary on National Sleep Foundation sleep quality recommendations." *Sleep Health* 2017;3:20-21.
    www.sciencedirect.com/science/article/pii/S2352721816301322?via%3 Dihub

12. Skarpsno ES, Mork PJ, Nilsen TIL, Holtermann A. "Sleep positions and nocturnal body movements based on free-living accelerometer recordings." *Nat Sci Sleep* 2017;9:267-275.
    www.ncbi.nlm.nih.gov/pmc/articles/PMC5677378/

13. Russo K, Bianchi MT. "How Reliable Is Self-Reported Body Position during Sleep?" *J Clin Sleep Med* 2015.
    www.ncbi.nlm.nih.gov/pmc/articles/PMC4702194/

14. Aserinsky E, Kleitman N. "Regularly occurring periods of eye motility, and concomitant phenomena, during sleep." *Science* 1953;118:273-274.
    https://neuro.psychiatryonline.org/doi/pdf/10.1176/jnp.15.4.454

15. MacFarlane AW. *Insomnia and its Therapeutics.* New York: William and Wood Company; 1891.

16. Dallaspezia S, Benedetti F. *Sleep deprivation as therapy in psychiatry.* In: Bianchi MT, ed. Sleep Deprivation and Disease. New York: Springer; 2014.

17. Consensus Conference P, Watson NF, Badr MS, et al. "Joint Consensus Statement of the American Academy of Sleep Medicine and Sleep Research Society on the Recommended Amount of Sleep for a Healthy Adult: Methodology and Discussion." *Sleep* 2015;38:1161-1183.
    www.ncbi.nlm.nih.gov/pmc/articles/PMC4507722/

18. Lavie P. "Self-reported sleep duration--what does it mean?" *J Sleep Res* 2009; 18:385-386.

19. Bliwise DL, Young TB. "The parable of parabola: what the U-shaped curve can and cannot tell us about sleep." *Sleep* 2007;30:1614-1615.
    www.ncbi.nlm.nih.gov/pmc/articles/PMC2276137/

20. Kurina LM, McClintock MK, Chen JH, Waite LJ, Thisted RA, Lauderdale DS. "Sleep duration and all-cause mortality: a critical review of measurement and associations." *Ann Epidemiol* 2013;23:361-370.
    www.ncbi.nlm.nih.gov/pmc/articles/PMC3660511/

21. Grandner MA, Patel NP, Gehrman PR, Perlis ML, Pack AI. "Problems associated with short sleep: bridging the gap between laboratory and epidemiological studies." *Sleep Med Rev* 2010;14:239-247.
    www.ncbi.nlm.nih.gov/pmc/articles/PMC2888649/

22. Leproult R, Deliens G, Gilson M, Peigneux P. "Beneficial impact of sleep extension on fasting insulin sensitivity in adults with habitual sleep restriction." *Sleep* 2015;38:707-715.
    www.ncbi.nlm.nih.gov/pmc/articles/PMC4402666/

23. Killick R, Hoyos CM, Melehan KL, Dungan GC, 2nd, Poh J, Liu PY. "Metabolic and hormonal effects of 'catch-up' sleep in men with chronic, repetitive, lifestyle-driven sleep restriction." *Clin Endocrinol (Oxf)* 2015;83:498-507.
    www.ncbi.nlm.nih.gov/pmc/articles/PMC4858168/

24. Tasali E, Chapotot F, Wroblewski K, Schoeller D. "The effects of extended bedtimes on sleep duration and food desire in overweight young adults: a home-based intervention." *Appetite* 2014;80:220-224.
    www.ncbi.nlm.nih.gov/pmc/articles/PMC4112413/

25. Lucassen EA, Piaggi P, Dsurney J, et al. "Sleep extension improves neurocognitive functions in chronically sleep-deprived obese individuals." *PLoS One* 2014;9:e84832.
    www.ncbi.nlm.nih.gov/pmc/articles/PMC3903365/

26. Alameddine Y, Ellenbogen JM, Bianchi MT. "Sleep-wake time perception varies by direct or indirect query." *J Clin Sleep Med* 2015;11:123-129. **www.ncbi.nlm.nih.gov/pmc/articles/PMC4298769/**

27. Fichten CS, Creti L, Amsel R, Bailes S, Libman E. "Time estimation in good and poor sleepers." *J Behav Med* 2005;28:537-553.

28. Miller CB, Gordon CJ, Toubia L, et al. "Agreement between simple questions about sleep duration and sleep diaries in a large online survey." *Sleep Health* 2015; 1:133–137.

29. Youngstedt SD, Goff EE, Reynolds AM, Khan N, Jeong M, Jean-Louis G. "Objective measures of sleep quality have not declined over the last 50 years." *Sleep Med Rev* 2016;30:108-109.

30. Horne J. *Sleeplessness: Assessing Sleep Need in Society Today.* Palgrave MacMillan; 2016.

31. Yetish G, Kaplan H, Gurven M, et al. "Natural sleep and its seasonal variations in three pre-industrial societies." *Curr Biol* 2015;25:2862-2868. **www.ncbi.nlm.nih.gov/pmc/articles/PMC4720388/**

32. Seymour JD, Fenley MA, Yaroch AL, Khan LK, Serdula M. "Fruit and vegetable environment, policy, and pricing workshop: introduction to the conference proceedings." *Prev Med* 2004;39 Suppl 2:S71-74.

33. Lin JS, O'Connor E, Whitlock EP, Beil TL. "Behavioral counseling to promote physical activity and a healthful diet to prevent cardiovascular disease in adults: a systematic review for the U.S. Preventive Services Task Force." *Ann Intern Med* 2010;153:736-750. **www.ncbi.nlm.nih.gov/pubmedhealth/PMH0009444/**

34. Vogel GW, Thurmond A, Gibbons P, Sloan K, Walker M. "REM sleep reduction effects on depression syndromes." *Arch Gen Psychiatry* 1975;32:765-777. **https://jamanetwork.com/journals/jamapsychiatry/fullarticle/491375**

35. Vogel GW. "Evidence for REM sleep deprivation as the mechanism of action of anti-depressant drugs." *Prog Neuropsychopharmacol Biol Psychiatry* 1983;7:343-349.

36. Grozinger M, Kogel P, Roschke J. "Effects of REM sleep awakenings and related wakening paradigms on the ultradian sleep cycle and the symptoms in depression." *J Psychiatr Res* 2002;36:299-308.

37. Ackermann S, Hartmann F, Papassotiropoulos A, de Quervain DJ, Rasch B. "No Associations between Interindividual Differences in Sleep Parameters and Episodic Memory Consolidation." *Sleep* 2015;38:951-959.
    www.ncbi.nlm.nih.gov/pmc/articles/PMC4434562/

38. Russo K, Goparaju B, Bianchi MT. "Consumer sleep monitors: is there a baby in the bathwater?" *Nat Sci Sleep* 2015;7:147-157.
    www.ncbi.nlm.nih.gov/pmc/articles/PMC4640400/

39. Ko PR, Kientz JA, Choe EK, Kay M, Landis CA, Watson NF. "Consumer Sleep Technologies: A Review of the Landscape." *J Clin Sleep Med* 2015;11:1455-1461.
    www.ncbi.nlm.nih.gov/pmc/articles/PMC4661339/

40. Bhat S, Ferraris A, Gupta D, et al. "Is There a Clinical Role For Smartphone Sleep Apps? Comparison of Sleep Cycle Detection by a Smartphone Application to Polysomnography." *J Clin Sleep Med* 2015;11:709-715.
    www.ncbi.nlm.nih.gov/pmc/articles/PMC4481053/

41. Behar J, Roebuck A, Domingos JS, Gederi E, Clifford GD. "A review of current sleep screening applications for smartphones." *Physiol Meas* 2013;34:R29-46.
    http://iopscience.iop.org/article/10.1088/0967-3334/34/7/R29/pdf

42. Accessed 5/17/2015, at http://mobihealthnews.com/43499/class-action-lawsuit-alleges-fitbit-misled-buyers-with-inaccurate-sleep-tracking/.

43. Ferini-Strambi L, Walters AS, Sica D. "The relationship among restless legs syndrome (Willis-Ekbom Disease), hypertension, cardiovascular disease, and cerebrovascular disease." *J Neurol* 2013.
    www.ncbi.nlm.nih.gov/pmc/articles/PMC4057632/

44. Walters AS, Rye DB. "Review of the relationship of restless legs syndrome and periodic limb movements in sleep to hypertension, heart disease, and stroke." *Sleep* 2009;32:589-597.
    www.ncbi.nlm.nih.gov/pmc/articles/pmid/19480225/

45. Lichstein KL, Justin Thomas S, Woosley JA, Geyer JD. "Co-occurring insomnia and obstructive sleep apnea." *Sleep Med* 2013;14:824-829.

46. Al-Jawder SE, Bahammam AS. "Comorbid insomnia in sleep-related breathing disorders: an under-recognized association." *Sleep Breath* 2012;16:295-304.

47. Luyster FS, Buysse DJ, Strollo PJ, Jr. "Comorbid insomnia and obstructive sleep apnea: challenges for clinical practice and research." *J Clin Sleep Med* 2010;6:196-204.
    www.ncbi.nlm.nih.gov/pmc/articles/PMC2854710/

48. Wickwire EM, Collop NA. "Insomnia and sleep-related breathing disorders." *Chest* 2010;137:1449-1463.

49. Van Dongen HP, Vitellaro KM, Dinges DF. "Individual differences in adult human sleep and wakefulness: Leitmotif for a research agenda." *Sleep* 2005;28:479-496.

50. Schutte-Rodin S, Broch L, Buysse D, Dorsey C, Sateia M. "Clinical guideline for the evaluation and management of chronic insomnia in adults." *J Clin Sleep Med* 2008;4:487-504.
    www.ncbi.nlm.nih.gov/pubmed/18853708

51. Alameddine Y, Klerman EB, Bianchi MT. *Caffeine and Naps as Countermeasures for Sleep Loss.* In: Bianchi MT, ed. Sleep Deprivation and Disease: Effects on the Body, Brain and Behavior: Springer; 2014.

52. Clark I, Landolt HP. "Coffee, caffeine, and sleep: A systematic review of epidemiological studies and randomized controlled trials." *Sleep Med Rev* 2017;31:70-78.

53. Sleep Hygiene. https://sleepfoundation.org/sleep-topics/sleep-hygiene.

54. Levenson JC, Kay DB, Buysse DJ. "The pathophysiology of insomnia." *Chest* 2015; 147:1179-1192.
    www.ncbi.nlm.nih.gov/pubmed/25846534

55. Trotti LM, Saini P, Koola C, LaBarbera V, Bliwise DL, Rye DB. "Flumazenil for the Treatment of Refractory Hypersomnolence: Clinical Experience with 153 Patients." *J Clin Sleep Med* 2016;12:1389-1394.
    www.ncbi.nlm.nih.gov/pmc/articles/PMC5033741/

56. Pavlova MK, Duffy JF, Shea SA. "Polysomnographic respiratory abnormalities in asymptomatic individuals." *Sleep* 2008;31:241-248.
    www.ncbi.nlm.nih.gov/pmc/articles/PMC2225571/

57. Sharma RA, Varga AW, Bubu OM, et al. "Obstructive Sleep Apnea Severity Affects Amyloid Burden in Cognitively Normal Elderly: A Longitudinal Study." *Am J Respir Crit Care Med* 2017.

58. Kapur VK, Auckley DH, Chowdhuri S, et al. "Clinical Practice Guideline for Diagnostic Testing for Adult Obstructive Sleep Apnea: An American Academy of Sleep Medicine Clinical Practice Guideline." *J Clin Sleep Med* 2017;13:479-504.
    www.ncbi.nlm.nih.gov/pubmed/28162150

59. Chervin RD, Aldrich MS. "The Epworth Sleepiness Scale may not reflect objective measures of sleepiness or sleep apnea." *Neurology* 1999;52:125-131.

60. Eiseman NA, Westover MB, Mietus JE, Thomas RJ, Bianchi MT. "Classification algorithms for predicting sleepiness and sleep apnea severity." *J Sleep Res* 2012; 21:101-112.
    www.ncbi.nlm.nih.gov/pmc/articles/PMC3698244/

61. Force USPST, Bibbins-Domingo K, Grossman DC, et al. "Screening for Obstructive Sleep Apnea in Adults: US Preventive Services Task Force Recommendation Statement." *JAMA* 2017;317:407-414.
    https://jamanetwork.com/journals/jama/fullarticle/2598778 (requires making account, but is free)

62. Moro M, Westover MB, Kelly J, Bianchi MT. "Decision Modeling in Sleep Apnea: The Critical Roles of Pretest Probability, Cost of Untreated Obstructive Sleep Apnea, and Time Horizon." *J Clin Sleep Med* 2016;12:409-418.
www.ncbi.nlm.nih.gov/pmc/articles/PMC4773629/

63. Bianchi MT, Goparaju B. "Potential Underestimation of Sleep Apnea Severity by At-Home Kits: Rescoring In-Laboratory Polysomnography Without Sleep Staging." *J Clin Sleep Med* 2017;13:551-555.
www.ncbi.nlm.nih.gov/pmc/articles/PMC5359331/

64. In: de Vries N, ed. Positional therapy in obstructive sleep apnea: Springer; 2014.

65. Ha SC, Hirai HW, Tsoi KK. "Comparison of positional therapy versus continuous positive airway pressure in patients with positional obstructive sleep apnea: a meta-analysis of randomized trials." *Sleep Med Rev* 2014;18:19-24.

66. Levendowski DJ, Seagraves S, Popovic D, Westbrook PR. "Assessment of a neck-based treatment and monitoring device for positional obstructive sleep apnea." *J Clin Sleep Med* 2014;10:863-871.
www.ncbi.nlm.nih.gov/pmc/articles/PMC4106940/

67. Boyd SB, Upender R, Walters AS, et al. "Effective Apnea-Hypopnea Index ("Effective AHI"): A New Measure of Effectiveness for Positive Airway Pressure Therapy." *Sleep* 2016;39:1961-1972.
www.ncbi.nlm.nih.gov/pmc/articles/PMC5070750/

68. Thomas RJ, Bianchi MT. "Urgent Need to Improve PAP Management: The Devil Is in Two (Fixable) Details." *J Clin Sleep Med* 2017;13:657-664.
www.ncbi.nlm.nih.gov/pmc/articles/pmid/28095974/

69. Ramar K, Dort LC, Katz SG, et al. "Clinical Practice Guideline for the Treatment of Obstructive Sleep Apnea and Snoring with Oral Appliance Therapy: An Update for 2015." *J Clin Sleep Med* 2015;11:773-827.
www.ncbi.nlm.nih.gov/pmc/articles/pmid/26094920/

70. Sateia MJ, Buysse DJ, Krystal AD, Neubauer DN, Heald JL. "Clinical Practice Guideline for the Pharmacologic Treatment of Chronic Insomnia in Adults: An American Academy of Sleep Medicine Clinical Practice Guideline." *J Clin Sleep Med* 2017;13:307-349.
    www.ncbi.nlm.nih.gov/pmc/articles/pmid/27998379/

71. Castillo J, Goparaju B, Bianchi MT. "Sleep-wake misperception in sleep apnea patients undergoing diagnostic versus titration polysomnography." *J Psychosom Res* 2014;76:361-367.
    www.ncbi.nlm.nih.gov/pmc/articles/pmid/24745776/

72. Harvey AG, Tang NK. "(Mis)perception of sleep in insomnia: A puzzle and a resolution." *Psychol Bull* 2012;138:77-101.
    www.ncbi.nlm.nih.gov/pmc/articles/PMC3277880/

73. Vgontzas AN, Fernandez-Mendoza J, Liao D, Bixler EO. "Insomnia with objective short sleep duration: The most biologically severe phenotype of the disorder." *Sleep Med Rev* 2013;17:241-254.
    www.ncbi.nlm.nih.gov/pmc/articles/PMC3672328/

74. Ekirch AR. *At day's close: night in times past.* 1st ed. New York: Norton; 2005.

75. Lichstein KL. "Insomnia identity." *Behav Res Ther* 2017;97:230-241.

76. FDA Drug Safety Communication: Risk of next-morning impairment after use of insomnia drugs. 2013. 2013, at /www.fda.gov/drugs/drugsafety/ucm334041.htm.)

77. Evaluating Drug Effects on the Ability to Operate a Motor Vehicle: Guidance for Industry. 2017. at www.fda.gov/ucm/groups/fdagov-public/@fdagov-drugs-gen/documents/document/ucm430374.pdf.)

78. Kripke DF. "Hypnotic drug risks of mortality, infection, depression, and cancer: but lack of benefit." *F1000Res* 2016;5:918.
    www.ncbi.nlm.nih.gov/pmc/articles/PMC4890308/

79. Morin CM, Vallieres A, Ivers H. "Dysfunctional beliefs and attitudes about sleep (DBAS): validation of a brief version (DBAS-16)." *Sleep* 2007;30:1547-1554.
www.ncbi.nlm.nih.gov/pmc/articles/PMC2082102/

80. Morgenthaler T, Kramer M, Alessi C, et al. "Practice parameters for the psychological and behavioral treatment of insomnia: an update. An american academy of sleep medicine report." *Sleep* 2006;29:1415-1419.

81. Espie CA, Luik AI, Cape J, et al. "Digital Cognitive Behavioural Therapy for Insomnia versus sleep hygiene education: the impact of improved sleep on functional health, quality of life and psychological well-being. Study protocol for a randomised controlled trial." *Trials* 2016;17:257.
www.ncbi.nlm.nih.gov/pmc/articles/pmid/27216112/

82. van der Zweerde T, Lancee J, Slottje P, et al. "Cost-effectiveness of i-Sleep, a guided online CBT intervention, for patients with insomnia in general practice: protocol of a pragmatic randomized controlled trial." *BMC Psychiatry* 2016;16:85.
www.ncbi.nlm.nih.gov/pmc/articles/PMC4818903/

83. Lancee J, van Straten A, Morina N, Kaldo V, Kamphuis JH. "Guided Online or Face-to-Face Cognitive Behavioral Treatment for Insomnia: A Randomized Wait-List Controlled Trial." *Sleep* 2016;39:183-191.
www.ncbi.nlm.nih.gov/pmc/articles/PMC4678352/

84. Cheng SK, Dizon J. "Computerised cognitive behavioural therapy for insomnia: a systematic review and meta-analysis." *Psychother Psychosom* 2012;81:206-216.

85. Pearson NJ, Johnson LL, Nahin RL. "Insomnia, trouble sleeping, and complementary and alternative medicine: Analysis of the 2002 national health interview survey data." *Arch Intern Med* 2006;166:1775-1782.

86. Bertisch SM, Wells RE, Smith MT, McCarthy EP. "Use of relaxation techniques and complementary and alternative medicine by American adults with insomnia symptoms: results from a national survey." *J Clin Sleep Med* 2012;8:681-691.
www.ncbi.nlm.nih.gov/pmc/articles/PMC3501665/

87. Brzezinski A, Vangel MG, Wurtman RJ, et al. "Effects of exogenous melatonin on sleep: a meta-analysis." *Sleep Med Rev* 2005;9:41-50.

88. Buscemi N, Vandermeer B, Hooton N, et al. "The efficacy and safety of exogenous melatonin for primary sleep disorders. A meta-analysis." *J Gen Intern Med* 2005;20:1151-1158.
    www.ncbi.nlm.nih.gov/pubmed/16423108

89. Bent S, Padula A, Moore D, Patterson M, Mehling W. "Valerian for sleep: a systematic review and meta-analysis." *Am J Med* 2006;119:1005-1012.
    www.ncbi.nlm.nih.gov/pmc/articles/PMC4394901/

90. Fernandez-San-Martin MI, Masa Font R, Palacios-Soler L, Sancho-Gomez P, Calbo-Caldentey C, Flores-Mateo G. "Effectiveness of Valerian on insomnia: a meta-analysis of randomized placebo-controlled trials." *Sleep Med* 2010;11:505-511.

91. Prasad VK, Cifu AS. *Ending Medical Reversal.* Johns Hopkins University Press; 2015.

92. Blendon RJ, DesRoches CM, Benson JM, Brodie M, Altman DE. "Americans' views on the use and regulation of dietary supplements." *Arch Intern Med* 2001;161:805-810.
    https://jamanetwork.com/journals/jamainternalmedicine/article-abstract /647749?redirect=true (requires making account, but is free)

93. Ashar BH, Rowland-Seymour A. "Advising patients who use dietary supplements." *Am J Med* 2008;121:91-97.
    http://www.sciencedirect.com/science/article/pii/S0002934307011369? via%3Dihub

94. Glisson JK, Walker LA. "How physicians should evaluate dietary supplements." *Am J Med* 2010;123:577-582.
    http://www.sciencedirect.com/science/article/pii/S0002934310000823? via%3Dihub

95. Newmaster SG, Grguric M, Shanmughanandhan D, Ramalingam S, Ragupathy S. "DNA barcoding detects contamination and substitution in North American herbal products." *BMC Med* 2013;11:222.
www.ncbi.nlm.nih.gov/pmc/articles/PMC3851815/

96. Zhou ES, Gardiner P, Bertisch SM. "Integrative Medicine for Insomnia." *Med Clin North Am* 2017;101:865-879.

97. Chang AM, Aeschbach D, Duffy JF, Czeisler CA. "Evening use of light-emitting eReaders negatively affects sleep, circadian timing, and next-morning alertness." *Proc Natl Acad Sci U S A* 2015;112:1232-1237.
www.ncbi.nlm.nih.gov/pmc/articles/PMC4313820/

98. Green A, Cohen-Zion M, Haim A, Dagan Y. "Evening light exposure to computer screens disrupts human sleep, biological rhythms, and attention abilities." *Chronobiol Int* 2017;34:855-865.

99. Zeitzer JM. "Real life trumps laboratory in matters of public health." *Proc Natl Acad Sci U S A* 2015;112:E1513.
www.ncbi.nlm.nih.gov/pmc/articles/PMC4386401/

100. Plante DT. "Leg actigraphy to quantify periodic limb movements of sleep: a systematic review and meta-analysis." *Sleep Med Rev* 2014;18:425-434.
www.ncbi.nlm.nih.gov/pmc/articles/PMC4135018/

101. Bianchi MT, Williams KL, McKinney S, Ellenbogen JM. "The subjective-objective mismatch in sleep perception among those with insomnia and sleep apnea." *J Sleep Res* 2013;22:557-568.
http://onlinelibrary.wiley.com/doi/10.1111/jsr.12046/epdf

102. Krueger JM, Frank MG, Wisor JP, Roy S. "Sleep function: Toward elucidating an enigma." *Sleep Med Rev* 2016;28:46-54.
www.ncbi.nlm.nih.gov/pmc/articles/PMC4769986/

103. Bianchi MT, Russo K, Gabbidon H, Smith T, Goparaju B, Westover MB. "Big data in sleep medicine: prospects and pitfalls in phenotyping." *Nat Sci Sleep* 2017;9:11-29.
www.ncbi.nlm.nih.gov/pmc/articles/PMC5317347/

104. Collop NA, Anderson WM, Boehlecke B, et al. "Clinical guidelines for the use of unattended portable monitors in the diagnosis of obstructive sleep apnea in adult patients. Portable Monitoring Task Force of the American Academy of Sleep Medicine." *J Clin Sleep Med* 2007;3:737-747.
www.ncbi.nlm.nih.gov/pmc/articles/PMC2556918/

105. Collop NA, Tracy SL, Kapur V, et al. "Obstructive sleep apnea devices for out-of-center (OOC) testing: technology evaluation." *J Clin Sleep Med* 2011;7:531-548.
www.ncbi.nlm.nih.gov/pmc/articles/PMC3190855/

106. Zinchuk AV, Gentry MJ, Concato J, Yaggi HK. "Phenotypes in obstructive sleep apnea: A definition, examples and evolution of approaches." *Sleep Med Rev* 2016.

107. Sands SA, Owens RL, Malhotra A. "New Approaches to Diagnosing Sleep-Disordered Breathing." *Sleep Med Clin* 2016;11:143-152.

108. Bianchi MT. "Screening for Obstructive Sleep Apnea: Bayes weighs in." *The Open Sleep Journal* 2009;2:56-59.
https://dash.harvard.edu/handle/1/23972578

109. Morgenthaler TI, Aurora RN, Brown T, et al. "Practice parameters for the use of autotitrating continuous positive airway pressure devices for titrating pressures and treating adult patients with obstructive sleep apnea syndrome: an update for 2007. An American Academy of Sleep Medicine report." *Sleep* 2008;31:141-147.
www.ncbi.nlm.nih.gov/pmc/articles/PMC2225554/

110. Morgenthaler T, Alessi C, Friedman L, et al. "Practice parameters for the use of actigraphy in the assessment of sleep and sleep disorders: an update for 2007." *Sleep* 2007;30:519-529.

111. Kolla BP, Mansukhani MP, Altchuler SI. "A Night of No Sleep?" *J Clin Sleep Med* 2016.
      www.ncbi.nlm.nih.gov/pmc/articles/PMC5155196/

112. Diekelmann S. "Sleep for cognitive enhancement." *Front Syst Neurosci* 2014;8:46.

113. **www.ncbi.nlm.nih.gov/pmc/articles/PMC3980112/**
      Dijk DJ. "Slow-wave sleep deficiency and enhancement: implications for insomnia and its management." *World J Biol Psychiatry* 2010;11 Suppl 1:22-28.

114. Bellesi M, Riedner BA, Garcia-Molina GN, Cirelli C, Tononi G. "Enhancement of sleep slow waves: underlying mechanisms and practical consequences." *Front Syst Neurosci* 2014;8:208.
      www.ncbi.nlm.nih.gov/pmc/articles/pmid/25389394/

115. Diekelmann S, Born J. "The memory function of sleep." *Nat Rev Neurosci* 2010;11: 114-126.

116. Marshall NS, Yee BJ, Desai AV, et al. "Two randomized placebo-controlled trials to evaluate the efficacy and tolerability of mirtazapine for the treatment of obstructive sleep apnea." *Sleep* 2008;31:824-831.
      www.ncbi.nlm.nih.gov/pubmed/18548827

117. Mason M, Welsh EJ, Smith I. "Drug therapy for obstructive sleep apnoea in adults." *Cochrane Database Syst Rev* 2013:CD003002.
      http://onlinelibrary.wiley.com/doi/10.1002/14651858.CD003002.pub3/ epdf/standard

118. Ulrich D. "Sleep Spindles as Facilitators of Memory Formation and Learning." *Neural Plast* 2016;2016:1796715.
      www.ncbi.nlm.nih.gov/pmc/articles/PMC4826925/

119. Manoach DS, Pan JQ, Purcell SM, Stickgold R. "Reduced Sleep Spindles in Schizophrenia: A Treatable Endophenotype That Links Risk Genes to Impaired Cognition?" *Biol Psychiatry* 2016;80:599-608.
      www.ncbi.nlm.nih.gov/pmc/articles/PMC4833702/

120. Bianchi MT. Essentials of sleep neuropharmacology. In: Barkoukis TJ, Matheson J, Ferber R, Doghramji K, eds. Therapy in Sleep Medicine: Elsevier; 2011.

121. Stein PK, Pu Y. "Heart rate variability, sleep and sleep disorders." *Sleep Med Rev* 2012;16:47-66.

122. Thomas RJ. "Sleep fragmentation and arousals from sleep-time scales, associations, and implications." *Clin Neurophysiol* 2006;117:707-711.

123. Bianchi MT, Thomas RJ. "Technical advances in the characterization of the complexity of sleep and sleep disorders." *Prog Neuropsychopharmacol Biol Psychiatry* 2013;45:277-286.
    www.ncbi.nlm.nih.gov/pmc/articles/PMC3631575/

124. Rechtschaffen A, Kales A. "A Manual of Standardized Terminology, Techniques, and Scoring System for Sleep Stages of Human Subjects." *(Washington, DC: US Government Printing Office)* 1968.

125. Silber MH, Ancoli-Israel S, Bonnet MH, et al. "The visual scoring of sleep in adults." *J Clin Sleep Med* 2007;3:121-131.

126. Van Dongen HP, Bender AM, Dinges DF. "Systematic individual differences in sleep homeostatic and circadian rhythm contributions to neurobehavioral impairment during sleep deprivation." *Accid Anal Prev* 2012;45 Suppl:11-16.
    www.ncbi.nlm.nih.gov/pmc/articles/PMC3260461/

127. Van Dongen HP, Belenky G. "Individual differences in vulnerability to sleep loss in the work environment." *Ind Health* 2009;47:518-526.
    www.jstage.jst.go.jp/article/indhealth/47/5/47_5_518/_pdf/-char/en

128. Friedman WA. "Resident duty hours in American neurosurgery." *Neurosurgery* 2004;54:925-931; discussion 931-923.

129. Philibert I, Nasca T, Brigham T, Shapiro J. "Duty-hour limits and patient care and resident outcomes: can high-quality studies offer insight into complex relationships?" *Annu Rev Med* 2013;64:467-483.

130. Milner CE, Cote KA. "Benefits of napping in healthy adults: impact of nap length, time of day, age, and experience with napping." *J Sleep Res* 2009;18:272-281.
      http://onlinelibrary.wiley.com/doi/10.1111/j.1365-2869.2008.00718.x/epdf

131. Zwyghuizen-Doorenbos A, Roehrs T, Timms V, Roth T. "Individual differences in the sedating effects of ethanol." *Alcohol Clin Exp Res* 1990;14:400-404.

132. Carney CE, Buysse DJ, Ancoli-Israel S, et al. "The consensus sleep diary: standardizing prospective sleep self-monitoring." *Sleep* 2012;35:287-302.

133. Sleep Diary. http://yoursleep.aasmnet.org/pdf/sleepdiary.pdf.

134. Quan SF, Budhiraja R, Clarke DP, et al. "Impact of treatment with continuous positive airway pressure (CPAP) on weight in obstructive sleep apnea." *J Clin Sleep Med* 2013;9:989-993.
      www.ncbi.nlm.nih.gov/pmc/articles/PMC3778188/

73383124R00099

Made in the
USA
Middletown, DE